Nursing and Midwifery in Britain since 1700

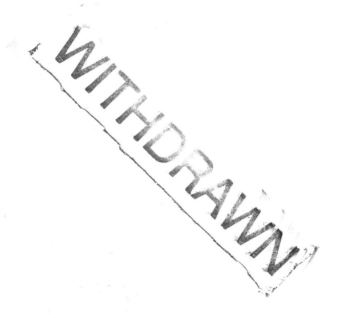

Nursing and Midwifery in Britain since 1700

Edited by

ANNE BORSAY AND BILLIE HUNTER

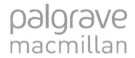

palgrave
macmillan

First published 2012 by
PALGRAVE MACMILLAN

Palgrave Macmillan in the UK is an imprint of Macmillan Publishers Limited, registered in England, company number 785998, of Houndmills, Basingstoke, Hampshire RG21 6XS.

Palgrave Macmillan in the US is a division of St Martin's Press LLC, 175 Fifth Avenue, New York, NY 10010.

Palgrave Macmillan is the global academic imprint of the above companies and has companies and representatives throughout the world.

Palgrave® and Macmillan® are registered trademarks in the United States, the United Kingdom, Europe and other countries.

ISBN 978–0–230–24703–1

This book is printed on paper suitable for recycling and made from fully managed and sustained forest sources. Logging, pulping and manufacturing processes are expected to conform to the environmental regulations of the country of origin.

A catalogue record for this book is available from the British Library.

A catalog record for this book is available from the Library of Congress.

10   9   8   7   6   5   4   3   2   1
21   20   19   18   17   16   15   14   13   12

Printed and bound in Great Britain by
CPI Antony Rowe, Chippenham and Eastbourne

Contents

Abbreviations

ACNM	American College of Nurse-Midwives
AIMS	Association for Improvements in Maternity Services
ARM	Association of Radical Midwives
ATNA	Australasian Trained Nurses' Association
BNA	British Nurses' Association
CMB	Central Midwives' Board
CMI	Catholic Maternity Institute
CNA	Canadian Nurses' Association
CNHS	Canadian National Health Service
DHSS	Department of Health and Social Security
DNHW	Department of National Health and Welfare
DRO	Devon Record Office
EMS	Emergency Medical Services
ERMH	Edinburgh Royal Maternity Hospital
EUL	Edinburgh University Library
FNS	Frontier Nursing Service
GMC	General Medical Council
GNC	General Nursing Council
GP	general practice
GPs	general practitioners
HMC	Hospital Management Committee
ICM	International Confederation of Midwives
IHS	Indian Health Service
LHSA	Lothian Health Services Archive
LOS	London Obstetrical Society (Although the Society preferred the name 'Obstetrical Society of London', the initials 'LOS' became the popular shorthand for both it and its midwifery examination and diploma, the only nationally recognized midwifery qualification before the 1902 Midwives Act.)
LSA	Local Supervising Authority
MANA	Midwives Alliance of North America
MH	Ministry of Health
MOH	Medical Officer of Health
Ms.	manuscript

MSL	Medical Society of London
NHS	National Health Service
NMC	Nursing and Midwifery Council
OHA	Oxfordshire Health Archives
QAIMNS	Queen Alexandra's Imperial Military Nursing Service
QNI	Queen's Nursing Institute
RAE	Research Assessment Exercise
RBNA	Royal British Nurses Association
RCM	Royal College of Midwives
RCN	Royal College of Nursing
RCPEd.	Royal College of Physicians, Edinburgh
RCSEng.	Royal College of Surgeons of England
RHB	Regional Health Board
RMC	Royal Maternity Charity
SEAN	State Enrolled Assistant Nurse
SEN	State Enrolled Nurse
SRN	State Registered Nurse
TWA	Tyne and Wear Archives
UKCC	United Kingdom Central Council for Nursing, Midwifery and Health Visiting (1983–2002)
VAD	Voluntary Aid Detachments
VON	Victorian Order of Nurses for Canada
Wellc.	Wellcome Library

Notes on Contributors

Anne Borsay is Professor of Healthcare and Medical Humanities in the College of Human and Health Sciences at Swansea University, UK.

Winifred Connerton is Postdoctoral Fellow at the Center for Health Outcomes and Policy Research and the Barbara Bates Center for the Study of the History of Nursing at the University of Pennsylvania School of Nursing, USA.

Patricia D'Antonio is Associate Professor of Nursing in the School of Nursing at the University of Pennsylvania, USA.

Christine E. Hallett is Professor of Nursing History in the School of Nursing, Midwifery and Social Work at the University of Manchester, UK.

Andrew Hull is Lecturer in the History of Medicine in the College of Human and Health Sciences at Swansea University, UK.

Billie Hunter is RCM Professor in Midwifery at the Cardiff School of Nursing and Midwifery Studies, Cardiff University, UK.

Andrea Jones held a PhD studentship between 2007 and 2010, funded by the Royal College of Nursing Wales, in the College of Human and Health Sciences at Swansea University, UK, where she researched nursing and political influence in Wales since 1948. She is now an oncology research nurse at Northampton General Hospital NHS Trust, UK.

Helen King is Professor of Classical Studies at the Open University, Milton Keynes, UK.

Alison Nuttall is Honorary Postdoctoral Fellow in the School of History, Classics and Archaeology at the University of Edinburgh, UK.

Anne Marie Rafferty is Professor of Nursing Policy in the School of Nursing and Midwifery at King's College London, UK.

Jane Sandall is Professor of Social Science and Women's Health in the Division of Women's Health in the School of Medicine at King's College London, UK.

1

Nursing and Midwifery: Historical Approaches

Anne Borsay and Billie Hunter

Health-care professionals have long recognized the significance of history for contemporary practice.[1] As early as 1921, for example, an article in the *British Journal of Nursing* insisted, 'No occupation can be quite intelligently followed or correctly understood unless it is, at least to some extent, illuminated by the light of history.' The nurse familiar with 'only her own time and surrounding' was 'unable to estimate and judge correctly the current events whose tendency is likely to affect her own career'. Therefore, it was essential to 'know how the work of nursing arose; what lines it has followed and under what direction it has best developed'.[2] Histories of nursing and midwifery have perpetuated the commitment to studying the past to improve the present. This is said to be especially useful at times of social change when practitioners struggle to assess new professional values[3] or come to terms with new political directives.[4] But learning from history is a complex process. As Nicky Leap and Billie Hunter found in their oral history of midwifery, there is no inevitable 'treasure chest of forgotten skills' to inspire today's midwives and enhance their practice; quite the opposite, prevailing attitudes were authoritarian.[5] Moreover, history never repeats itself; contrary to popular opinion, 'nothing in human society ... ever happens twice under exactly the same conditions or in exactly the same way'. Consequently, though drawing analogies or parallels between the past and the present may deepen our understanding of current problems, it is unlikely to offer simple solutions.[6]

1

So is it mistaken to see relevance in the history of nursing and midwifery? Not at all! In recent years, multidisciplinary working and the reconfiguration of roles have seriously challenged traditional professional identities. At the same time, confidence is being shaken by economic uncertainties, the political dilemmas of trade union action and the social reverberations of shifting gender, class and ethnic relations. Therefore, neither nurses nor midwives are any longer 'ascribed a single identity by virtue of their ... occupational group'. Instead, they are compelled 'to construct their own identities on an ongoing basis by thrashing out the multiple meanings of their changing roles'.[7] *Nursing and Midwifery in Britain since 1700* is designed to contribute to the critical reflection that such identity-building requires, by illustrating how historical analysis can help to compile professional narratives that explore present-day experiences with reference to the past.

Origins

The words 'nurse' and 'midwife' passed into the English language during the Middle Ages: a long period in British history, which stretched for a thousand years from the departure of the Romans in the fifth century to the arrival of the Tudor monarchy in 1485. 'Nurse' – derived from the Latin *nutricius* or *nutritius*, meaning 'to nourish' – became 'norse' or 'nurice'.[8] 'Midwife' – derived from the Anglo-Saxon – was translated as 'with-woman', meaning the midwife herself and not the mother.[9] In the early medieval period, the boundaries between nursing and midwifery and between medicine and obstetrics were permeable and the division of labour less gendered than it is today. From the twelfth century, however, the barring of women from the universities, and from the guilds that governed surgeons and apothecaries in towns, slowly eroded their formal healing roles if not their domination of family and community medicine.[10] Midwifery fared better than nursing. Therefore, in her study of *Women's Healthcare in the Medieval West*, Monica Green chose to include midwives but exclude nurses from the list of health-care practitioners. Whereas midwifery had a clearly identifiable role around the autonomous care of mothers and babies, the 'modern, quite specific professional medical connotations of "nurse" ... [had] no place in the Middle Ages'. As a result, she decided, it was 'best to restrict the term to those women ... [usually children's nurses] who were so designated in medieval documents'.[11]

The well-defined modern nurse who serves as Green's benchmark is a figment of the imagination. By the time the verb 'to nurse' and the noun 'nursing' joined the person of 'the nurse' in the sixteenth century, the meaning of all three terms had broadened to include the tending and nourishment of inanimate objects such as land and money as well as the care of patients of all ages.[12] However, exactly what that care entailed remained far from certain. Therefore, when Florence Nightingale – Britain's most famous nurse, renowned for her exploits during the Crimean War (1853–6) – published *Notes on Nursing* in 1859, she acknowledged that nursing was not well understood:

> I use the word nursing for want of a better. It has been limited to signify little more than the administration of medicines and the application of poultices. It ought to signify the proper use of fresh air, light, warmth, cleanliness, quiet, and the proper selection and administration of diet – all at the least expense of vital power to the patient.[13]

Twentieth-century nurses continued to emphasize their jurisdiction over this distinctive healing environment, regarded as essential for effective medical diagnosis and treatment. The focus thus fell on 'patients as whole beings' rather than as the victims of specific diseases; and well-being was construed as not just 'physical intactness' but also as 'emotional and social integration'.[14] By the 1960s, nursing was beginning to collaborate more directly with medicine, moving towards a role that demanded 'independence of thought and action'.[15] However, there is no greater clarity about its definition. As the authors of the recent *History of the Royal College of Nursing* (RCN) conclude, 'The answer to the question . . . "what is the proper task of a nurse", remains open.' Too many groups describe themselves as nurses. Therefore, it is impossible for the profession to secure its position, as medicine and midwifery have done, by exhibiting command of a unique body of knowledge and skills.[16]

For some historians of nursing and midwifery, this preoccupation with professional status is a distraction. In 1996, for instance, Christopher Maggs made a powerful case for advancing beyond 'the discipline of the technologies' – 'that of medicine or nursing or physiotherapy' or indeed midwifery – and developing 'a history of caring . . . to cross over all of the disciplines which contribute to health'.[17] To date his call has gone largely unheeded. Outside the modern period during which nurses and midwives established their professional credentials, studies have looked at caring in families and local communities. But post-1800, the drive towards professionalization has eclipsed this perspective and research has concentrated on themes such as the battle for registration, the debate about trade unionism and models of organization, education and training.[18] Nevertheless, the historical analysis of these issues has not stood still. In response to broader historiographical trends, it has evolved from hagiographic celebration at the end of the nineteenth century into an energetic area of scholarship dedicated to locating nursing and midwifery within their economic and political, social and cultural contexts.

Histories

The history of nursing and midwifery has its roots in Victorian biography, which praised the lives of 'women worthies' as exemplars for female readers.[19] At the Midwives' Institute, four women were particularly prominent between the 1880s and 1914 as the organization campaigned to achieve registration and promote the expertise of its members: Zepherina Smith, Jane Wilson, Amy Hughes and Rosalind Paget. Though Paget has been described as 'the Florence Nightingale of midwifery',[20] her work failed to generate the biographical interest provoked by nursing's 'lady with a lamp'. Nightingale herself wrote on maternal mortality and midwifery training following an outbreak of puerperal sepsis in 1867 which led to the closing down of her school for midwives at King's College Hospital in London.[21] However, such failures were of no concern to early biographers such as Sarah Tooley, whose romantic *Life* – published in 1904 to mark the 50th anniversary of Florence's departure to the Crimea – was an unadulterated celebration of womanly self-sacrifice.[22]

Over the course of the twentieth century, the genre of *critical* biographies emerged,[23] and in their later studies of Nightingale neither Sir Edward Cook[24] nor Cecil Woodham-Smith[25] indulged in Tooley's brand of personality whitewash. Until the late 1990s,[26] however, Nightingale's performance at the Scutari Military Hospital during the Crimean War remained untarnished. Mark Bostridge destroyed this orthodoxy in a pungent piece on the BBC's history webpage. Historians, he argued, were only just

> waking up to the shocking truth that the death toll at Nightingale's hospital was higher than at any other hospital in the East, and that her lack of knowledge of the disastrous sanitary conditions at Scutari was responsible. 4,077 soldiers died at Scutari during Nightingale's first

winter there, ten times more from illnesses such as typhus, typhoid, cholera and dysentery, than from battle wounds. Conditions at the hospital were fatal to the men that Nightingale was trying to nurse: they were packed like sardines into an unventilated building on top of defective sewers.[27]

Bostridge's assessment is more restrained in his seminal biography of Nightingale, where he concedes that 'the dramatic decrease in mortality at Scutari in the first months of 1855' was 'directly attributable' to her.[28] Nevertheless, it was the sanitary commission, despatched by the British government six months after Nightingale's arrival, which significantly cut the mortality rate by flushing out the sewers and improving ventilation. And only while preparing evidence for the Royal Commission on the Health of the Army did Florence herself realize that she had helped soldiers 'to die in cleaner surroundings and greater comfort, but she had not saved their lives'.[29]

Such critical biographies have many virtues as a historical tool, bringing people to life and enabling neglected figures to rise from obscurity. Exemplary in this respect is Jane Robinson's rehabilitation of the black nurse, Mary Seacole[30] – quickly forgotten after her death, but greeted with 'rapturous enthusiasm' at the public banquet held in London to honour Crimean soldiers.[31] Nevertheless, biographies do overlook the everyday lives of ordinary nurses and midwives, not to mention the patients for whom they cared. One way of broadening the focus is to look at the institutions through which the two professions evolved. Early institutional histories were as eulogistic as early biographies, making little attempt to dig beneath the surface and question achievements or acknowledge shortcomings.[32] But even in contemporary studies, there is a tendency to exaggerate. Susan Williams may thus be a little bullish in asserting that the 1936 Midwives' Act, which set up a national salaried midwifery service, was an achievement of the National Birthday Trust Fund.[33] Moreover, institutional histories tend to gravitate towards the 'big names'. Therefore, the recent RCN study noted: 'Although the views of its leaders were undoubtedly influenced by changing climates of opinion, and shifts in social and gender relations, they were also active in contributing to some of these changes.' It followed that 'due weight' had to be given to 'the role of... [the organization's] leaders, not as a celebratory "institutional history", but to explain how an organization of this type survives, and how it adjusts to new circumstances'.[34]

Given the tenor of personal and institutional biographies, the past experiences of both nurses and midwives also need to be situated within their broader historical context. This call for context underpins Sioban Nelson's 'fork in the road': the division between nursing and midwifery histories, which tells a story of progress from 'the dark and chaotic past to the glorious present'; and *histories of* nursing and midwifery, which engage with mainstream historical scholarship by addressing the complex economic, social, political and cultural environments in which nurses and midwives worked.[35] The implementation of context was both empirical and conceptual. In the history of nursing, empiricism – the belief in evidential as opposed to theoretical or logical justification – was pioneered by Brian Abel-Smith, whose *A History of the Nursing Profession* was published in 1960.[36] Abel-Smith examined the politics of general nursing, paying particular attention to the role of structure, recruitment, terms and conditions, professional associations and trade unions. As Christine Hallett says, he 'deliberately challenged the progressive perspective by revealing... the tensions and conflicts which existed within the nursing establishment'; the 'profession's leaders' were 'No longer a group of noble women driving towards the same goal,... [but] fallible... fractured... [and] capable of sabotaging as well as promoting... [their] own interests.'[37]

The history of midwifery has also attracted empirical investigation. In his monumental study of *Death in Childbirth* between 1800 and 1950, Irvine Loudon tested 'the effectiveness of various forms of maternal care by means of the measurement of maternal mortality'. His nuanced conclusion was that 'high maternal risk could be associated with cheap untrained midwives or expensive over-zealous and unskilled doctors'. On the other hand, 'Sound obstetric practice by well-trained midwives could produce low levels of maternal mortality even in populations that were socially and economically deprived.' 'Monocausal explanations' of these patterns were criticized, given the potential influence of 'clinical or pathological factors', 'social and economic changes', 'the politics of maternal care' and 'the quality of medical education'. But, equally, social-historical and feminist accounts 'with scarcely a statistic, let alone a statistical evaluation, in sight' were severely chastised. For if demography detracted 'attention from features of central importance which are inherently unmeasurable – attitudes or sentiments for example – there... [was] also the danger that without statistical analysis large conclusions are often based on the shaky foundation of thin evidence and small unrepresentative samples'.[38]

Abel-Smith was more apologetic about missing the essence of professional practice, admitting that nursing as 'an activity or skill' – and 'what it was like ... to nurse ... or to receive nursing care' – was largely absent from his picture.[39] Monica Baly started to fill these gaps in the first edition (1973) of *Nursing and Social Change*. For her, 'The development of nursing ... [was] like weaving a cloth with social change as the warp, and running to and fro with the weft ... [was] the shuttle of care.'[40] Yet although the endorsement of contextualization was unequivocal, Baly's narrative retained the progressive ethos. From the late 1970s, this confidence was shaken as the forces attributed with determining the economic, social and political structures of modern societies since the late eighteenth century – the nation state, industrialization, social class, science and religion – were dethroned by economic crisis, industrial conflict, faltering political institutions and procedures and a virulent attack on public services.[41] The result was a collapse of the consensus built around the welfare state, which had emerged post-1945 in the aftermath of the Second World War.[42] This crisis set the stage for nursing sociologist Celia Davies to attack the supposition that 'progressive and humanitarian ideas ... [would] eventually win out against the opposition of vested interests'. No, this was not the case. Reforms were 'double-edged, always in part at least reflecting the views of the most powerful'.[43] It was this assault on the inevitability of progress, derived from a background in the social sciences, which supplied the history of nursing with its conceptual toolkit for the analysis of context.

Midwifery as well as nursing is closely aligned with the social sciences, using them to oppose 'the alleged positivistic and technocratic values of medicine'.[44] Consequently, concepts derived from the social sciences have been a friendly medium for historical contextualization. This new orientation has encouraged research forays into patient interests[45] and the employment of overseas nurses,[46] but most activity has concentrated on gender and labour histories.[47] Although both nursing and midwifery are predominantly female professions, the concept of gender has been differentially employed. In the history of nursing, the organization of nineteenth-century hospitals has been explained in terms of domestic patriarchy, with the 'doctor/nurse relationship' becoming 'the man–father/women–mother relationship' and being 'subsumed under the rubric of male–female relations'.[48] Furthermore, it has been suggested that at times of war, these gendered roles are destabilized,[49] nowhere more so than when the 'nurse entered into a direct physical relationship with the wounded soldier'.[50] But, otherwise, surprisingly little attention has been paid to gender issues.

The history of midwifery, on the other hand, has embraced gender more enthusiastically. Confrontation with the predominantly male medical profession for the control of childbirth may account for this difference. Midwives have used history to track the 'medical takeover' of their role which, allegedly, gathered momentum after the introduction of ante-natal care in the early twentieth century and peaked in the 1970s with the acceleration of hospital births. It has been argued that midwifery 'belong[ed] to a woman's world where instinct, intuition and emotion as well as clinical competence and theoretical knowledge play their parts'. Therefore, routine hospitalization and the indiscriminate use of technology have not only threatened midwives' careers but have also reduced pregnancy and childbirth to a 'mechanistic exercise' for women.[51] More recent histories have been cautious about the decline of midwifery, stressing diversity rather than uniformity. As Hilary Marland and Anne Marie Rafferty concluded after reviewing the chapters in their edited collection, midwives' practice is a product of not only the 'development of the obstetric professions' and 'levels of institutional provision' but also of 'economic forces, urbanization, changes in family life and the employment of women, religion . . . [and] the input . . . of various pressure groups'.[52]

In labour history too, similar refinement has taken place. Sociologist Mick Carpenter is one of a few people who have taken an interest in nursing from an employment perspective. Characterizing how nurses became professionalized in Britain, Carpenter identified 'three main attempted transformations'. Nightingale's name was attached to the first phase, which 'lasted from the mid-nineteenth century to around the time of the First World War' and tried to establish an autonomous 'nursing structure', despite 'subordination' to 'the managerial needs of the local hospital' and to medicine. The second phase – 'the professionalization of care' – was 'initiated in the late nineteenth century by Mrs Bedford Fenwick'. Its mission was to achieve the 'social closure' of nursing 'as an exclusively middle class occupation' by seeking professional independence from 'the state and local managements', by extending the control of 'general nursing over the nursing universe' and by attaining a 'complementary' (though 'still subordinated position') in relation to 'an ascendant medicine'. The third phase – 'the new professionalism' – crossed the Atlantic to Britain in the 1970s and was predicated on a 'renewed' effort 'to achieve the longstanding goals of professionalization'.

But 'whereas previous movements . . . sought to professionalize the whole occupation', the new professionalism concentrated on clinical nurses, aiming to provide them with a knowledge base – separate from medicine – that challenged biomedicine in the name of the patient by developing nursing plans that were 'rational, rigorous and individualized'.[53]

Professionalization has dominated the histories of both nursing and midwifery, as the chapters in this volume demonstrate. In her 2005 Monica Baly Lecture, however, Celia Davies issued a plea to 'ditch' the concept of professionalization in favour of a 'professional identity', which was better able to absorb the complexities of 'nursing knowledge, practice, regulation and caring'.[54] This call is now being answered. Building on Christopher Maggs's pioneering study of nurse recruitment at four provincial hospitals,[55] Sue Hawkins has continued the task of unpicking the stereotypical images of nineteenth-century nursing and providing the historical detail to hone sociological models such as that of Carpenter. Using St George's Hospital, London, as a case study, she has shown that although there was some movement towards the reformers' ideal of the young unmarried nurse from the higher social classes, working-class women had not been excluded from hospital nursing by 1900. Moreover, far from being 'the docile, saintly nurse of myth', they had taken a positive and informed decision to enter the profession as a career choice within a labour market that was offering women an increasing number of options.[56]

This contextualization of nurses within an economic environment is indicative of a wider maturity in the history of nursing and midwifery. So too is the broadening of focus beyond the fortunes of general nursing to encompass both hospital specialties[57] and community services.[58] The trend away from 'an internalist and triumphalist form of professional apologetics to a robust and reflective area of scholarship' – noted by the editors of *Nursing History and the Politics of Welfare* in 1997 – has been consolidated.[59]

Doing History

The transition of scholarship in the history of nursing and midwifery was underpinned by a lively debate about sources and methods. When established as an academic discipline during the nineteenth century, history embraced the rational pursuit of objective truth in line with the mindset of the natural sciences; in the words of the German historian Leopold von Ranke, it sought 'to show how, essentially, things happened'.[60] From the 1970s, however, the economic and political decline that undermined faith in progress also threatened intellectual confidence in objectivity, emphasizing the relativity of knowledge and reducing it to power. 'We should admit . . . that power produces knowledge', declared the French philosopher Michel Foucault, 'that knowledge and power directly imply one another'.[61] Accordingly, the past could not be understood in a rational way, because every interpretation was merely the outcome of political values. Yet while this postmodern approach has provoked vibrant debate about the nature of history,[62] it has never been more than a marginal force in Britain, with some impact on the range of sources that historians deploy but little on the methods that they use to construct historical arguments.

Given the affinity of nursing and midwifery with the social sciences, it is not surprising that the histories of the two professions have emphasized the different source bases; whereas social scientists design a project to collect the data required, historians generally have to work with what has survived.[63] Until recently, they used to rely almost exclusively on documentary evidence. Inevitably, there are problems. Documents can be damaged or destroyed, for example; there may be major gaps in their coverage; and, in the case of eighteenth-century nursing, references are few and far between because nurses were only slowly forming as an occupational group. Striving for a robust methodology, historians ask three key questions: Is this source what it says it is? Who wrote it? And for what purposes?[64] The history of nursing and midwifery is no exception. Therefore, the chapters in this volume will call heavily on sources such as government papers (e.g. Acts of Parliament, government reports, criminal records from courts such as the Old Bailey and statistical series such as the ten-yearly Census and infant and maternal mortality rates); materials relating to non-state institutions (in particular, the rules, annual reports, minute books and casebooks for hospitals, charities and professional organizations); nursing, midwifery and medical books; advice literature for patients; professional journals; lecture notes for students; diaries and correspondence; and trade directories and advertisements.

Complementing these documentary sources is oral history. Originating in ancient songs and legends passed on by word of mouth, oral sources were later rejected as incompatible with the scientific mentality of the discipline. Their revival was facilitated in the 1960s by the rise of social history, its potential for more democratic, socially conscious research resonating with the decade's egalitarian ethos. Of course, there are drawbacks. Only recent history is accessible, dates may be uncertainly remembered, meanings may be reconstituted over time and stereotypical social roles may be reproduced. But the capacity of oral history to rescue groups missing from the written record and to correct distorted images makes it an invaluable tool for the history of nursing and midwifery.[65] Some studies were informally conducted, penetrating uncharted territory. In Lindsay Reid's collection of 20 testimonies from Scottish midwives, for instance, Joan Spence, who trained in 1970, recalled how:

> The wee chap came out and he was grossly deformed. His limbs were all round the wrong way. I ran out of the room with him and I ran into a paediatrician. The baby was barely alive. The paediatrician wanted to take him from me and resuscitate him but he died within minutes. The poor woman, I've never forgotten her. I don't think she ever saw that baby again.[66]

Sweet and Dougall's systematic oral histories – one element within their investigation of twentieth-century community nursing – are equally revealing on subjects as sensitive as inter-professional relations; for example, one narrator described the district nurse and the health visitor as 'like you know chalk and cheese' before the introduction of general practice (GP) attachments in the 1970s.[67]

The source base has been further expanded by the way in which postmodernism has eroded the importance attached to society's economic, social and political structures and hence created the potential for artefacts, visual imagery and imaginative literature to shape – and not just reflect – historical experience.[68] Consequently, these media have become sources to which at least some historians resort. In the history of nursing and midwifery, as in the discipline as a whole, extracting the meaning of artefacts such as the nurse's uniform or the midwife's bag is a struggle in which few have as yet participated.[69] Visual imagery – paintings, photographs, films and television – and imaginative literature – novels, drama, poetry – are also underexploited, history failing to follow the example of literary studies.[70] Therefore, it would be a mistake to exaggerate the effects of postmodernism on history's commitment to documentary sources. What has happened, however, is their more inventive deployment.

In her study of nursing periodicals, Elaine Thomson grasped the new agenda by understanding their advertising as a way to 'structure the meaning for products and commodities'. As she explains:

> advertisements aimed at nurses form a discursive space where definitions of femininity, and of professional roles and identities, are endorsed

and reproduced. They tell us much about the aspirations of the nurse, the way she was perceived – by herself and others – and her place in medicine and in society.[71]

New information technologies have also enabled the pioneering treatment of documentary sources. In this spirit, Sue Hawkins has broken new ground with her prosopographical methodology. Undaunted by the lack of letters and diaries regarded as essential for biographical projects, she set about building a database of nurses at St George's Hospital in London between 1850 and 1900. Nurse registers, wage books and minute books were scrutinized, together with the *Census*, *The Hospital* and *Nursing Record*, and a mid-1890s survey of matrons in the capital. It was with these data that she was able to substantiate the continued presence of working-class women in the nursing community.[72]

The postmodern critique of objectivity served to remind historians that such sources offered no straightforward access to the past. However, it is important not to exaggerate the novelty of this warning. Firstly, the traditional interrogation of documentary material had always confronted the question of what had motivated the production of sources. Secondly, from the early 1960s, some historians had challenged the feasibility of objective knowledge, insisting that writings about the past were coloured both by the personal characteristics of their authors – social class, race, gender, age, politics – and by the contemporary societies in which they lived.[73] Therefore, the management of different interpretations of the same phenomenon was an integral part of historical analysis. In 1996, Angela Cushing attempted to reassert the case for objective methods in the history of nursing, maintaining that historical explanation was an 'inductive' process in which general arguments were inferred from particular instances or 'facts'; it was 'not a mere interpretation of the texts provided by the people of the past'.[74] Though her article stimulated heated debate in the *International History of Nursing Journal*,[75] the matter of objectivity has not been entirely resolved. Thus in their recent *Notes on Nightingale*, Sioban Nelson and Anne Marie Rafferty still found it necessary to urge 'an awareness of the nuances of historical scholarship and the complexity of the past, as opposed to seeing it as a set of "facts"'.[76]

Nursing and midwifery history is not alone in resisting the implications of postmodernism. Yet if knowledge is informed by power[77] and the search for one objective truth is misguided, it remains possible to pursue 'a multiplicity of accurate histories' whose divergence is an engine for exciting intellectual exchange.[78] So how do we do accurate history? There is now a splendid array of general texts supplying detailed guidance on how to read historical sources[79] and apply them to the shaping of historical analysis.[80] Moreover, the history of nursing and midwifery has also acquired relevant chapters and articles.[81] At a mechanical level, the use of footnotes for referencing sources and the work of other authors allows each point to be checked and evaluated. But it is in the process of writing that the historian gets to grips with the competing interpretations that make objectivity unrealistic.

Writing involves constructing arguments by making claims based on primary sources, deploying concepts and theories and engaging with other accounts, drawn from the historical literature.[82] Social science techniques such as discourse analysis are superficially attractive for this task. However, the minute way in which they examine texts means that 'it is imperative to have a limited body of data with which to work',[83] whereas research in history proceeds by identifying as wide a spectrum of sources as possible and placing them within their broad context. More useful is the way in which social scientists have conceptualized analysis as consisting of two complementary processes: 'the segmenting of data into relevant categories' and the reassembling of these data when 'the categories are related to one another to generate theoretical understanding'.[84] This exercise has been dismissed as an 'anecdotal approach' in which 'the representativeness or generality of... [the] fragments is rarely addressed'.[85] But in history, as in qualitative social research, the goal is not validation in the scientific sense. Rather, credibility grounded in 'structural corroboration' is sought, where 'the researcher relates multiple types of data to support or contradict the interpretation'.[86] It is a 'feat... only accomplished as a result of much trial and error'.[87]

Using This Book

The enthusiasm of nurses and midwives for understanding the past is displayed in the personal recollections and historical series that have long graced the professional journals.[88] During the 1970s, for example, *Midwife and Health Visitor* ran a long series called 'History and Progress', which traced the development of a wide variety of health-care practices. Our review of histories, sources and methods in this chapter has shown that the assumption of progress – however deep-seated – is an untenable one. In the chapters that follow, we attempt to demonstrate why. The research base for this endeavour is variable, not only because sources may be fragmented, but also because much activity was London-based and the provinces and Scotland, Wales and Ireland have been neglected. Moreover, the chronological demands of the project have led us to privilege the general nurse over the specialist nurse and the hospital over the community – 'the key battleground for the various forces arrayed in the division of labour in health care'.[89] But for the first time since the path-breaking *An Introduction to the Social History of Nursing* was published in 1988,[90] we offer a long-range history of nursing and midwifery.

The book has five distinctive features. First, it brings together both professions on an equal footing, rather than limiting the coverage of midwifery and implying that it is a subsidiary of nursing. Second, it looks beyond the recent past, opening in 1700 and surveying the long eighteenth century to 1830, rather than taking for granted that nothing of any moment took place before the early nineteenth century. Third, though unable to do full justice to the international dimension,[91] it presents a comparative assessment of Britain's global sphere of influence in Australia, the United States and Canada. Fourth, the similarities and differences that have characterized and shaped the two professions are teased out. And, finally, a short epilogue explores the implications of the historical analysis for contemporary policy and practice.

Imposing a standardized format on this agenda, spanning two professions over three centuries, would threaten its historical integrity. However, six main themes in addition to professionalization recur throughout the book: the locus of care; gender, class and ethnicity; the emergence of specialisms; and interprofessional relations between nursing, midwifery and medicine. The six chapters (Chapters 2–7) on British nursing and midwifery between 1700 and 2000 conclude by relating their content to these themes. In this way, we put forward a co-ordinated history of nursing and midwifery.

You can approach the volume in several ways: by reading it from cover to cover, by focusing only on nursing or midwifery and by looking at each profession chronologically – in other words, by tackling Chapters 2 and 5, Chapters 3 and 6 and Chapters 4 and 7 together. Whatever method you chose, we hope that the book will act as a stimulus for future study and research.

Notes

1. This chapter develops themes raised in Anne Borsay's 2006 Monica Baly Lecture, a revised version of which was subsequently published as 'Nursing History: An Irrelevance for Nursing Practice?', *Nursing History Review*, 17 (2009) 14–27.
2. 'Why We Study Nursing History', *British Journal of Nursing*, 66 (5 February 1921) 79.
3. R. White, *Social Change and the Development of the Nursing Profession: A Study of the Poor Law Nursing Service, 1848–1948* (London: Henry Kimpton Publishers, 1978) p. 2.
4. J. Towler and J. Bramall, *Midwives in History and Society* (London: Croom Helm, 1986) Foreword.
5. N. Leap and B. Hunter (eds), *The Midwife's Tale: An Oral History from Handywoman to Professional Midwife* (London: Scarlet Press, 1993) pp. xi, 193.
6. J. Tosh, *The Pursuit of History: Aims, Methods and New Directions in the Study of Modern History*, 2nd edn (London: Longman, 1991) pp. 10–22.
7. Borsay, 'Nursing History', 21.
8. L. Whaley, *Women and the Practice of Medical Care in Early Modern Europe, 1400–1800* (Basingstoke: Palgrave Macmillan, 2011) p. 113.
9. J. Donnison, *Midwives and Medical Men: A History of the Struggle for the Control of Childbirth*, 2nd edn (London: Historical Publications, 1988) p. 11; E. Duff, 'Wisdom, Skill, Companionship, Earth, Life, the Kneeling Woman: The Meaning of Midwife', *MIDIRS Midwifery Digest*, 18:1 (2008) 55.
10. M. Connor Versluysen, 'Old Wives' Tales? Women Healers in English History', in C. Davies (ed.), *Rewriting Nursing History* (London: Croom Helm, 1980) pp. 175–89; V.L. Bullough and B. Bullough, 'Medieval Nursing', *Nursing History Review*, 1 (1993) 89–101.
11. M.H. Green, *Women's Healthcare in the Medieval West: Texts and Contexts* (Aldershot: Ashgate, 2000) p. 341.
12. S. Donaghue, 'Humanist Traditions in Nursing Development', *The Australian Nurses' Journal*, 4 (1975) 27.
13. F. Nightingale, *Notes on Nursing: What It Is and What It Is Not*, 1st edn 1860 (Edinburgh: Churchill Livingstone, 1980) p. 2.
14. C.E. Hallett, *Containing Trauma: Nursing Work in the First World War* (Manchester: Manchester University Press, 2009) pp. 2–3.
15. E. Pearce, *General Textbook of Nursing*, 17th edn (London: Faber, 1967) p. 21; E. Pearce, *General Textbook of Nursing*, 20th edn (London, Faber, 1980) p. xvii. We are grateful to Andrew Hull for these references.
16. S. McGann, A. Crowther and R. Dougall, *A History of the Royal College of Nursing, 1919–1999: A Voice for Nurses* (Manchester: Manchester University Press, 2009) p. 325.

17. C. Maggs, 'Towards a History of Nursing', *International History of Nursing Journal*, 1:4 (1996) 90.
18. C. Maggs, 'A History of Nursing: A History of Caring?', *Journal of Advanced Nursing*, 23 (1996) 632.
19. J. Purvis, 'From "Women Worthies" to Poststructuralism? Debate and Controversy in Women's History in Britain', in J. Purvis (ed.), *Women's History: Britain, 1850–1945* (London: UCL Press, 1995) pp. 1–2.
20. J. Hannam, 'Rosalind Paget: The Midwife, the Women's Movement and Reform before 1914', in H. Marland and A.-M. Rafferty (eds), *Midwives, Society and Childbirth: Debates and Controversies in the Modern Period* (London: Routledge, 1997) pp. 83–6.
21. P.M. Dunn, 'Florence Nightingale (1820–1910): Maternal Mortality and the Training of Midwives', *Archives of Disease in Childhood*, 74 (1996) 219–20.
22. S. Tooley, *A Life of Florence Nightingale* (London: S.H. Bousfield, 1904).
23. See, for example, B. Caine, *Biography and History* (Basingstoke: Palgrave Macmillan, 2010).
24. E. Cook, *The Life of Florence Nightingale*, 2 vols (New York: Macmillan, 1913).
25. C. Woodham-Smith, *Florence Nightingale, 1820–1910* (London: Constable, 1950).
26. For an early revisionist account, see H. Small, *Florence Nightingale: Avenging Angel* (London: Constable, 1998).
27. M. Bostridge, 'Florence Nightingale: The Lady with the Lamp', BBC Online History, http://www.bbc.co.uk/cgi-bin/history/rende ... discovery/medicine/nightingale_myth1.shtm, accessed 23 September 2001.
28. M. Bostridge, *Florence Nightingale: The Woman and Her Legend* (London: Viking, 2008) p. 249.
29. M. Bostridge, 'Florence Nightingale'.
30. J. Robinson, *Mary Seacole: The Charismatic Black Nurse Who Became a Heroine of the Crimea* (London: Constable, 2005).
31. 'Mary Seacole, 1805–1881', *Medi Theme*, 25:3 (2006) 98.
32. See, for example, E. Bendall and E. Raybould, *A History of the General Nursing Council for England and Wales, 1919–1969* (London: H.K. Lewis, 1969); B. Cowell and D. Wainwright, *Behind the Blue Door: The History of the Royal College of Midwives, 1881–1981* (London: Bailliere Tindall, 1981); M. Stocks, *A Hundred Years of District Nursing* (London: Allen and Unwin, 1960).
33. A.S. Williams, *Women and Childbirth in the Twentieth Century: A History of the National Birthday Trust Fund, 1928–1993* (Stroud: Sutton Publishing, 1997) Dustjacket.
34. McGann, Crowther and Dougall, *History*, p. 3.
35. S. Nelson, 'The Fork in the Road: Nursing History versus the History of Nursing?', *Nursing History Review*, 10 (2002) 175–6.

36. B. Abel-Smith, *A History of the Nursing Profession* (London: Heinemann, 1960).
37. C. Hallett, 'Century of Transformation? Historical Perspectives on Nineteenth-Century Nursing', *Women's History Magazine*, 65 (2011) 4–5.
38. I. Loudon, *Death in Childbirth: An International Study of Maternal Care and Maternal Mortality, 1800–1950* (Oxford: Clarendon Press, 1992) pp. 5–6, 517.
39. Abel-Smith, *History*, p. xi.
40. M. Baly, *Nursing and Social Change*, 3rd edn (London: Routledge, 1995) p. xiii.
41. A. Munslow, *Deconstructing History* (London: Routledge, 1997) pp. 14–15.
42. For an overview of post-war British history, see P. Clarke, *Hope and Glory: Britain, 1900–1990* (London: Penguin, 1996) Chapters 7–11; D. Kavanagh and P. Morris, *Consensus Politics from Attlee to Thatcher* (Oxford: Blackwell, 1989).
43. C. Davies, 'Introduction: The Contemporary Challenge in Nursing History', in C. Davies (ed.), *Rewriting Nursing History* (London: Croom Helm, 1980) p. 12.
44. A.M. Rafferty, 'Writing, Researching and Reflexivity in Nursing History', *Nurse Researcher*, 5:2 (Winter 1997/98) 5–16.
45. R. Hawker, 'For the Good of the Patient?', in C. Maggs (ed.), *Nursing History: The State of the Art* (London: Croom Helm, 1987) pp. 143–52.
46. M. Shkimba and K. Flynn, ' "In England We Did Nursing": Caribbean and British Nurses in Great Britain and Canada, 1950–70', in B. Mortimer and S. McGann (eds), *New Directions in the History of Nursing: International Perspectives* (London: Routledge, 2005), pp. 141–57.
47. S. Hawkins, *Nursing and Women's Labour in the Nineteenth Century: The Quest for Independence* (London: Routledge, 2010) p. 8.
48. E. Gamarnikow, 'Women's Employment and the Sexual Division of Labour: The Case for Nursing', in A. Kuhn and A. Wolpe (eds), *Feminism and Materialism: Women and Modes of Production* (London: Routledge and Kegan Paul, 1978) p. 111.
49. M.R. Higonnet and P.L.R. Higonnet, 'The Double Helix', in M.R. Higonett (ed.), *Behind the Lines: Gender and the Two World Wars* (New Haven: Yale University Press, 1987) p. 35.
50. A. Summers, *Angels and Citizens: British Women as Military Nurses, 1854–1914* (London: Routledge and Kegan Paul, 1988) p. 273.
51. Towler and Bramall, *Midwives*, p. ix.
52. H. Marland and A.M. Rafferty, 'Introduction', in Marland and Rafferty (eds), *Midwives*, p. 5.
53. M. Carpenter, 'The Subordination of Nurses in Health Care: Towards a Social Divisions Approach', in E. Riska and K. Wegar (eds), *Gender,*

Work and Medicine: Women and the Medical Division of Labour (London: Sage, 1993) pp. 115–25.

54. H. Sweet, 'And Our Own Conference . . .', *History Info: Newsletter of the Royal College of Nursing History of Nursing Society* (Winter 2005/6) 8.

55. C. Maggs, *The Origins of General Nursing* (London: Croom Helm, 1983).

56. Hawkins, *Nursing*, pp. 32, 56, 171, 182.

57. See, for example, S. Kirby, 'Sputum and the Scent of Wallflowers: Nursing in Tuberculosis Sanatoria, 1920–1970', *Social History of Medicine*, 23:3 (2010) 602–20.

58. See, for example, H.M. Sweet with R. Dougall, *Community Nursing and Primary Healthcare in Twentieth-Century Britain* (Abingdon: Routledge, 2008).

59. 'Introduction', in A.M. Rafferty, J. Robinson and R. Elkan (eds), *Nursing History and the Politics of Welfare* (London: Routledge, 1997) p. 1.

60. J. Warren, *The Past and Its Presenters: An Introduction to Issues in Historiography* (London: Hodder and Stoughton, 1998) p. 104.

61. M. Foucault, *Discipline and Punish: The Birth of the Prison*, trans. A. Sheridan (Harmondsworth: Penguin, 1977) p. 27.

62. See, for example, K. Jenkins, *Re-thinking History* (London: Routledge, 1991); R.J. Evans, *In Defence of History* (London: Granta Books, 1997).

63. Rafferty, 'Writing', p. 2 (online version).

64. A. Marwick, *The Nature of History* (London: Macmillan, 1970) pp. 136–7.

65. For appraisals of oral history, see P. Thompson, *The Voice of the Past* (Oxford: Oxford University Press, 1978); R. Perks and A. Thomson (eds), *The Oral History Reader*, 2nd edn (London: Routledge, 2006); B. Roberts, *Biographical Research* (Buckingham: Open University Press, 2002) Chapter 6, pp. 93–114.

66. L. Reid, *Scottish Midwives: Twentieth-Century Voices* (East Linton, East Lothian: Tuckwell Press, 2000) p. 173.

67. Sweet with Dougall, *Community Nursing*, p. 92.

68. S.L. Gilman, *Health and Illness: Images of Difference* (London: Reaktion Books, 1995) pp. 9–20.

69. A.D. Hood, 'Material Culture: The Object', in S. Barber and C.M. Peniston-Bird (eds), *History beyond the Text: A Student's Guide to Approaching Alternative Sources* (Abingdon: Routledge, 2009) pp. 176–98.

70. J. Hallam, *Nursing the Image: Media, Culture and Professional Identity* (London: Routledge, 2000); A. Hudson Jones (ed.), *Images of Nurses: Perspectives from History, Art and Literature* (Philadelphia: University of Pennsylvania Press, 1988).

71. E. Thomson, ' "Beware of Worthless Imitations": Advertising in Nursing Periodicals, *c*.1888–1945', in Mortimer and McGann (eds), *New Directions* (London: Routledge, 2005), pp. 158–9.

72. Hawkins, *Nursing*, pp. 9–10. See also M. Damant, 'A Biographical Profile of Queen's Nurses in Britain, 1910–1968', *Social History of Medicine*, 23:3 (2010) 586–601.

73. E.H. Carr, *What Is History?* (Harmondsworth: Penguin, 1961) p. 8.

74. A. Cushing, 'Method and Theory in the Practice of Nursing History', *International History of Nursing Journal*, 2:2 (1996) 13.

75. See, for example, C. Maggs, 'A Response to Angela Cushing', *International History of Nursing Journal*, 2:2 (1996) 88–91; A. Cushing, 'Method and Theory in the Practice of Nursing History', *International History of Nursing Journal*, 2:4 (1997) 58–63; C. Holmes, 'History, Interpretation and Social Theory: A Personal Rejoinder', *International History of Nursing Journal*, 3:1 (1997) 30–43.

76. S. Nelson and A.M. Rafferty, 'Introduction', in S. Nelson and A.M. Rafferty (eds), *Notes on Nightingale: The Influence and Legacy of a Nursing Icon* (New York: Cornell University Press, 2010) p. 5.

77. A. Borsay, 'Medical Records as Catalogues of Experience', in M. Evans and I.G. Finlay (eds), *Medical Humanities* (London: BMJ Books, 2001) pp. 56–7.

78. J. Appleby, L. Hunt and M. Jacob, *Telling the Truth about History* (New York: W.W. Norton, 1994) pp. 261–2.

79. Barber and Peniston-Bird (eds), *History beyond the Text*; M. Dobson and B. Ziemann (eds), *Reading Primary Sources: The Interpretation of Texts from Nineteenth- and Twentieth-Century History* (London: Routledge, 2009) pp. 159–74.

80. See, for example, L. Jordanova, *History in Practice* (London: Arnold, 2000); Tosh, *Pursuit of History*.

81. See, for example, J. Foster and J. Sheppard, 'Archives and the History of Nursing', in Davies (ed.), *Rewriting*, pp. 200–14; L.A. Hall, 'Nurses in the Archives: Archival Sources for Nursing History', in Rafferty, Robinson and Elkan (eds), *Nursing History*, pp. 259–73; J. Sweeney, 'Historical Research: Examining Documentary Sources', *Nurse Researcher*, 12:3 (2005) 61–73; J. Allotey, 'Writing Midwives' History: Problems and Pitfalls', *Midwifery*, 27:2 (2011) 131–7.

82. Jordanova, *History*, pp. 185–6.

83. D. Silverman, *Interpreting Qualitative Data: Methods for Analysing Talk*, 3rd edn (London: Sage, 2006) pp. 194–5. See also L. Prior, *Using Documents in Social Research* (London: Sage, 2003).

84. H. Boeije, *Analysis in Qualitative Research* (London: Sage, 2010) p. 76.

85. A. Bryman, *Quantity and Quality in Social Research* (London: Unwin Hyman, 1988) p. 77.

86. J.W. Cresswell, *Qualitative Inquiry and Research Design: Choosing among Five Approaches*, 2nd edn (Thousand Oaks, California: Sage, 2007) p. 204.

87. Tosh, *Pursuit*, p. 110.

88. J.E. Gordon, 'Nurses and Nursing in Britain: 7. The Hospital Tradition from the Reformation to the Eighteenth Century', *Midwife and Health Visitor*, 6 (December 1970) 457–62; H. Arthure, 'Midwifery Practice in the First Half of the Twentieth Century', *Midwife, Health Visitor and Community Nurse*, 11 (October 1975) 333–4. See also I. McMillan, 'Insight into Bedlam: One Hospital's History', *Journal of Psychosocial Nursing*, 35:6 (1997) 28–34.
89. R. Dingwall, A.M. Rafferty and C. Webster, *An Introduction to the Social History of Nursing* (London: Routledge, 1988) p. 228.
90. Dingwall, Rafferty and Webster, *Introduction*.
91. See, for example, B. Mortimer and S. McGann (eds), *New Directions in the History of Nursing: International Perspectives* (London: Routledge, 2005); Marland and Rafferty (eds), *Midwives*.

PART I

NURSING 1700–2000

In the first part of this book, the history of nursing in Britain between 1700 and 2000 is examined in three chronological stages.

In Chapter 2: *Nursing, 1700–1830: Families, Communities, Institutions,* Anne Borsay considers the origins of the profession. Although nurses only emerged as a professional group in the late nineteenth century, significant developments that helped to shape their modern role occurred during the long eighteenth century, which stretched from 1700 until the 1820s. Nursing took place in domestic, community and institutional settings. Domestic assistance for relatives, friends and neighbours and community care offered privately or under the Poor Law were by far the most common, but institutional nursing was much more visible. There were several types of institution, but this chapter focuses on voluntary hospitals for the acute sick. Wild tales of drunken and disorderly nurses are exaggerated. Hospitals sought a caring attitude, and while nurses undertook domestic tasks, there is also evidence that they attended to the bodily and clinical needs of patients.

Chapter 3: *Nursing, 1830–1920: Forging a Profession* by Christine E. Hallett continues the story of change post-1830. The author explains how the private nurse and the hospital nurse were joined by the English nursing sisterhoods, whose vocational and religious emphases later influenced the development of the profession. The 'reforms' of the nineteenth century are assessed with reference to professionalization and the influence of Florence Nightingale. The importance of military nursing is recognized through the Queen Alexandra's Imperial Military Nursing Service (QAIMNS); and the wartime participation of British nurses is examined with reference to the 'volunteer-nurse' and especially the 'rise of the VAD' during the First World War. Finally, the author traces the 'professionalizing project' of the late nineteenth and early twentieth centuries, taking into account the formation of the Royal British Nurses Association (RBNA) in 1887, the establishment of the three earliest nursing journals and the setting up of the Royal College of Nursing (RCN) in 1916.

In Chapter 4: *Nursing 1920–2000: The Dilemmas of Professionalization*, by Andrew Hull with Andrea Jones, the challenge of professionalization in the twentieth century is explored. The authors identify the educational and managerial strategies that were used by nursing leaders to increase the status of nurses and tease out how these ideas came into conflict with the demand for cheap labour. Before the birth of the National Health Service (NHS) in 1948, the matron was responsible for all aspects of nursing in her hospital, including the education of nurses. In the aftermath of the NHS, however, her role was gradually fragmented. There was a brief reprieve during a phase of consensus management when matrons rejoined other healthcare professions and enjoyed renewed influence due to the size of the nursing budget. But with the appointment of business managers in the 1980s, the matron receded and professionalization was once more pursued by developing separately the educational qualifications and managerial skills of nurses. The authors analyse how the quest for professionalization was underpinned by ideological differences about the role of the nurse and the nature of nursing.

The chapters in this part provide insights into the origins of nursing and its subsequent development and professionalization. These insights should be borne in mind when reading the 'sister' chapters in Part II, which consider the history of midwifery over the same period. There are similarities and differences in the evolution of both professions. Both have engaged in similar professional projects, with education and research seen as the means to achieving professional status, and both have had to manage the challenge of being gendered occupations. There are differences, however, in how these professional projects have been played out. The chapters in this first part illustrate how the development of a diverse range of nursing roles and specialties, together with the persistence of conflicting understandings of the unique function of the nurse, has presented challenges for the professionalization of nursing. As will be seen, these concerns differ from those experienced by midwives.

2

Nursing, 1700–1830: Families, Communities, Institutions

Anne Borsay

> She was a fat old woman, this Mrs Gamp, with a husky voice and
> a moist eye, which she had a remarkable power of turning up, and
> only showing the white of it. Having very little neck, it cost her some
> trouble to look over herself, if one may say so, at those to whom she
> talked. She wore a very rusty black gown, rather the worse for snuff,
> and a shawl and bonnet to correspond.[1]

Sarah Gamp, the disreputable nurse in Charles Dickens' novel, *Martin
Chuzzlewit*, haunts the history of pre-Nightingale nursing. Yet published in the 1840s as part of Dickens' propaganda campaign for
social reform,[2] this image bears little resemblance to those who practiced during the long eighteenth century. These nurses were part of
a diverse collection of healers and supporters. In families and local
communities, folklore and accumulated experience informed dietary
and herbal remedies often based on the contents of larders and gar-
dens.[3] To this informal repertoire were added medical practitioners,
defined as 'any individual whose occupation is basically concerned
with the care of the sick'.[4] Therefore, health care was the preserve
not only of physicians, surgeons, and apothecaries or druggists who
had attended university or followed apprenticeships but also of midwives, itinerant healers, mountebanks who sold patent medicines and
'wise women' who on occasions trod a fine line with witchcraft.[5]

The purpose of Chapter 2 is to explore the role of nursing within this matrix, focusing on domestic households, local communities and institutions. It will argue that professionalization had its roots not in the Nightingale era but in the voluntary hospitals of the previous century.

Domestic Nursing

Domestic nursing, ministering to relatives, servants and the local community, remained vibrant up to 1830, and was recognized as a cost-effective and accessible means of care and treatment. Medical practitioners endorsed this input, working in concert with lay healers and only periodically raising their voices against unsupervised medication. Ginnie Smith has argued that the humoral system of medicine facilitated this collaboration because it 'constituted a science of nursing'[6] in which good health was attributed to a set of environmental factors (air, diet, exercise, weather) interacting with a bodily constitution where the humours (blood, phlegm, yellow bile and black bile) were in equilibrium. Derived from the ancient Greek principles of Hippocrates, this theory generated recommendations for lifestyle changes and purgative therapies that were consistent with lay practice.[7] Therefore, humoralism preserved the integration of nursing and doctoring that had characterized health care in the centuries before 1700.

Many of the remedies used by domestic nurses were orally transmitted from generation to generation, but some were transcribed in written manuscripts,[8] and by the early eighteenth century printed health literature was expanding the repertoire of the literate who could afford the price. Given its long association with small children, it is not surprising that nursing achieved coverage in these texts on the coat-tails of child care. In the 1740s, for example, the physician William Cadogan published *An Essay upon the Nursing and Management of Children, from Their Birth to Three Years of Age*.[9] Volumes by other physicians specializing in child care followed. It was in 1774, however, that Dr Hugh Smith first published his *Letter to Married Women on Nursing and the Management of Their Children*.[10]

Whereas Cadogan – as physician to the London Foundling Hospital for abandoned children – had addressed his text to one of the governors, Smith wrote for women themselves and chose 'the familiar style of letter-writing' as the 'most eligible' way of communicating his message. The *Letter* was significant in two respects. First, as in *The*

Family Physician of 1773, Smith extended nursing from children to adults, arguing that both successful child care and 'preserving infirm and aged constitutions' were heavily dependent upon the good nurse. Second, he specified nursing's relationship to medicine, insisting that it was 'of first consequence' in rearing infants, curing diseases, and 'preserving . . . delicate and feeble constitutions'. 'For although, by the medical art, many violent and dangerous diseases may oftentimes be prevented from proving fatal; yet, even when the doctor has taken his leave, the good nurse must still be watchful to restore again the invalid to a healthy and vigorous constitution.'[11]

Despite linking adult and child nursing, the bulk of Smith's *Letter* was devoted to pregnancy and child care. Nevertheless, some advice on the care of older patients was offered. In addition to barring inappropriate visitors from the sick room, the good nurse was to ensure clean linen and the free circulation of air; serve 'a proper, light, and nourishing diet'; dispense medication punctually; and 'seek the assistance of able and experienced physicians'. Yet though urged 'to alleviate bodily infirmities' by supporting the patient's spirit, she was given no guidance on the nursing skills required for these tasks. The reason was an elision of nursing with women's family responsibilities, underpinned by the assumption that they possessed the requisite skills. In the 'sick chamber', Smith declared, 'the conjugal affection of a wife is laudably displayed – the tender love of a mother fondly exerts itself – the gratitude and duty of a daughter are conspicuous – the good sister also endears herself to a worthy brother – and female friendship wears a thousand additional charms!'[12]

We cannot assume polarized gender roles from this advice literature, with men occupying the public world of work and politics and women occupying the private world of the home. On the contrary, women in the upper and middle classes were active in consumerism, property-holding and philanthropy, while the emphasis on caring was later used by feminist writers to press the case for women's unique contribution to the state.[13] Furthermore, presiding over a system of domestic health care that not only embraced doctoring as well as nursing but also took in servants, employees and the local community as well as relatives was in itself a source of power and influence. As George Woodward, vicar of East Hendred near Wantage in Berkshire, proudly reported in correspondence with an uncle in 1760: 'Agues are much about, and my wife . . . has multitude of patients, that come to her three or four miles round, and great success she has with her powders.'[14]

Community Nursing

Domestic health care among the lower orders is less easily disaggregated from community nursing because the Poor Law authorities supported family care, paying relatives to live with elderly people[15] and 'making allowances to parents when children were sick... [in] recognition that nursing them involved real opportunity costs'.[16] Non-relatives were also reimbursed for caring. In the north Wales parish of Towyn, for example, Humphrey David was paid weekly for the 'diet and nursing' of three poor neighbours, all of them women. Moreover, he was still providing the same service a decade later.[17] Additional to these parish nurses were handywomen, private nurses and charitable nurses working in the community. The online edition of *The Proceedings of the Old Bailey* has opened up the everyday lives of ordinary people like nurses who left relatively few other traces. Published between 1674 and 1913, the *Proceedings* record trials for crimes committed in London and Middlesex. They cannot be used for quantitative analysis or to track changes over time for two reasons: the collection of trials is incomplete, particularly for the early eighteenth century; and although not significantly distorted, the transcripts are a partial version of events. Trivial offences like small value thefts are only briefly reported, for instance; and the case for the defence is often abridged and prosecution evidence occasionally omitted.[18] Furthermore, in interpreting testimonies, the reliability of alleged criminals and witnesses cannot be assumed. Nevertheless, searching with the terms 'nurse', 'nurses' and 'nursing' does enable us to build up a qualitative picture of what nurses did, which extends beyond the criminal justice system to their often irretrievable caring roles.

The *Proceedings* confirm a place for the handywoman. Deborah Sheene, found not guilty of theft from her employer in 1795, was thus described as undertaking 'any handy work that a woman can do, she quilts petticoats, and she has been nursing sick people'.[19] However, the traditional distinction between handywoman and private nurse was far from rigid. The private nurse in a wealthy household may have been restricted to nursing, but in less well-off households there were similarities to the handywoman. Martha Nicholls, summoned as a prosecution witness to a burglary in 1798, explained that she was a nurse to the victim's wife and 'was there after she was dead to wash the things up'.[20] As well as dealing with death, nurses combined domestic duties with their caring role, Ann Edwards having been a servant for two years 'as a nurse and chamber maid' when she was transported for stealing from her employer in 1752.[21] Elizabeth Davies, employed by William Smith in 1828 'to nurse my wife, and to do domestic work', implied an intimate relationship with the family when she claimed that 'Mrs Smith knew of my pawning the things, to get various little things which Mr Smith did not allow her, grapes, pastry, and liquor.' The court unconvinced sentenced her to four months in prison.[22]

Although the *Proceedings* typically mention nurses and nursing in only general terms, the occasional references to patient groups indicate that a variety of cases were handled. Private nurses complemented the role of midwives, looking after women before and after the birth of their babies,[23] and caring for children.[24] Infectious diseases were managed in both children and adults,[25] but nurses also dealt with long-term chronic conditions. Jane Chapman, prosecution witness at a trial for theft in 1796, nursed a single woman called Elizabeth Yeoman, who had 'lost the use of her limbs almost a year and an half';[26] while in 1826 Hannah Green received the death penalty for stealing money from her patient, Amelia Bund, who was 'confined to . . . bed with a paralytic stroke'.[27] Mental illness as well as physical disabilities were tended. In 1750 Sarah Privinix testified at William Archer's trial for murder that she was 'nurse in the house when anything ailed him; he was so mad about nine years ago, he was corded down in his bed, and I have known him to be as mad as any man in Bedlam [a London asylum], three times within this Twelvemonth'.[28]

Parish and charitable nurses were visible via their employing organizations. Poor Law records disclose that parish nursing was not an exclusively female occupation. In the Bedfordshire parish of Campton, for example, Samantha Williams found that between 1767 and 1834 16 per cent of the 'carers' recruited to supply paupers with domestic and nursing assistance were men. However, whereas women 'undertook the full range of task work, most of the male carers were paid on odd occasions just to attend other men'. In comparison to the early eighteenth century, there may have been a reduction in the medical activities performed by both genders,[29] as the spiralling cost of poor relief forced a concentration on basic care.[30] Nevertheless, their roles did include the management of serious injuries. When Richard Parrott, subsequently convicted of murder in 1761, cut out his wife's tongue, for example, Mary Dew was 'desired' by the 'officers of the parish' to nurse her. As she told the court, 'I staid a week with her, she was very much swelled, and her mouth very much abused; I poulticed it, and brought it down, and put plaisters of brown paper and treacle to her throat.'[31] But it was the engagement of parish nurses with child care that was most controversial.

In 1716, a Parliamentary Committee, set up to investigate the funding of London poor relief, reported: 'That a great many poor infants, and exposed bastard children, are inhumanly suffered to die by the barbarity of nurses, especially parish nurses, who are a sort of people void of commiseration, or religion.' In St Martin-in-the-Fields, for instance – allegedly one of the more successful parishes – over three-quarters of the infants cared for by nurses died each year. Though reviled as child murderers, nurses were – like their charges – victims of a parsimonious Poor Law system which, as the Parliamentary Committee recognized, sought the cheapest rates 'to take off a burthen from the parish'.[32] The plight of London's children, allied to concerns about population decline, led to the emergence of a fourth group of 'country' or charitable nurses employed by the Foundling Hospital after it was established by charitable subscription in 1739. Most of the women were recruited from counties adjacent to the capital. On arrival in London, they were examined for infectious diseases, their milk supply was checked and they were given clothing and simple medicines for the child, and taught how to wean. On returning home, they were subjected to the surveillance of inspectors, drawn primarily from the clergy, minor gentry and substantial tradesman. And as a result, the mortality rate halved.[33]

In her 1925 study of London, Dorothy George concluded that the nursing of infants and children 'progressively improved' from the 1750s.[34] The evidence is too slight to pass this judgement on any branch of community nursing. Throughout the eighteenth century, some nurses were recruited via the workhouse, indicative of their vulnerable, impoverished or even disreputable backgrounds.[35] Convictions, notably for theft from employers, also continued.[36] But the Old Bailey *Proceedings* also show nurses acting as respected members of the community. In 1741, when Christopher Shotton had been on trial for murdering a fellow player during a cricket match, Ann Foster told the court that while nursing him after his injury:

> He had a violent Fever and Convulsions, and all his Complaint was of his left Side, so that he could not lie upon it. I used to ask him his Complaint, and he said those Rogues that beat one have killed me, and hang them, hang them: These were his Words. I saw him open'd, and he was all black on the Heart, and one of his Ribs was broke . . . [37]

Community nurses gave character references as well as medical evidence. In 1744 a parish nurse called Elizabeth Ball was instrumental in the acquittal of Ann Collier for highway robbery. 'I have known her between two and three years,' she testified, 'and never say anything amiss of her.'[38]

Institutional Nursing

Although eighteenth-century community nursing was less abject than conventional wisdom alleges, it was the institution that saw the first steps towards professionalization. Nurses were employed in five main types of institution: prisons, military establishments, workhouses, asylums and hospitals. Little is known about prison nursing.[39] In military establishments, on the other hand, nursing was integral to patient care. At the Chelsea Hospital – one of two institutions founded by the monarchy towards the end of the seventeenth century for elderly and disabled veterans – Ann Grant had a detailed knowledge of James Legg's mental health, which she put forward when he was tried for the murder of another pensioner. Having nursed him for nine years, she 'saw a very great change ...; a lowness, a melancholy and deranged state'. He told her that 'his mind was confused; that he had no rest night or day; that he was hurried from place to place, and could not tell what he was doing'. But despite being afraid that he would commit suicide or 'do himself an injury', she never raised these concerns with a doctor because she thought he was 'harmless'.[40] It is unlikely that the women who – contrary to popular opinion – nursed men on active service functioned with the same degree of autonomy, given the presence of military doctors. Nonetheless, Sir John Pringle recognized a distinctive nursing role in his 1753 *Observations on the Diseases of the Army*; and a decade later eighteen nurses, together with two head nurses and a matron, were recruited from hospitals in Britain to staff military hospitals abroad during the Seven Years' War against Spain.[41]

Hospitals were one of three types of domestic medical institution, the other two being workhouses and asylums. Workhouses developed within the framework of the 1601 Poor Law, which primarily supported the 'deserving' elderly, sick or 'infirm' within the community. However, as Jeremy Boulton has demonstrated, parish nurses in London were running *de facto* nursing homes for the sick poor from the 1690s until halted by the metropolitan workhouse movement in the first quarter of the eighteenth century.[42] Nationwide, Poor Law authorities were permitted after 1723 to restrict able-bodied assistance to the workhouse, but institutional populations remained mixed and it was 60 years before new legislation decreed that only those 'indigent by old age, sickness or infirmities' should be sent to the workhouse.[43] In arguing that, under this system, 'the sick were looked after by the other inmates' with no special provision,[44] Rosemary White overlooks the significance of workhouse policy for nursing. True, paupers were responsible for sick inmates and their integrity was not always copper-bottomed, the theft of workhouse sheets to pawn proving a particular temptation.[45] Like Ann Hudson at the St Giles' Workhouse in London, however, they were 'employed as a nurse' and hence recruited into an identifiable role.[46] Moreover, like community nurses, some institutional nurses were regarded as sufficiently upstanding citizens to give evidence in court. In 1732 Mary Davis thus testified that while putting Richard Percival to bed in St James' Workhouse, he told her that he had been wounded while 'playing the Rogue with a Man about a piece of Bread and Butter. That he fell back, and coming forward again, the Prisoner stab'd him in the Belly. He died about 8 in the morning.'[47]

Whereas the workhouse was a general-purpose institution, asylums were dedicated to mental illness and learning difficulty – impairments known by a variety of contemporary terms from 'insanity' and 'madness' to 'idiocy' and 'stupidity'. The first asylum was the famous Bethlem Hospital in London, a monastic foundation dating back to the medieval period. By the early eighteenth century, this foundation had been joined by fee-paying or commercial institutions and by charitable institutions, funded by a single benefactor or by public subscription.[48] The first documented employment of a nurse at Bethlem occurred in 1692, but her brief was the treatment of physical illness and the job was abandoned as 'a separate office' in 1765. In the same year, matrons – in post from at least the early seventeenth century but only allocated housekeeping jobs – became responsible for the female wards, much as the steward oversaw the male wards. Duties included ensuring that the patients were kept clean and their 'Straw . . . changed when Damp or Dirty'; requiring those who were capable of employment not to be idle; informing the physician when they stayed in bed 'without particular Sickness'; and where necessary removing the sick to the infirmary, albeit an inadequate one. The routine care of patients was under the control of keepers, who until 1815 were called 'basketmen' after the receptacles in which the medieval brothers had collected donations of food.[49]

At the York Retreat, opened by the Society of Friends in 1796, the title of attendant was adopted for the male staff who supervised male patients; female patients were cared for by female nurses, although 'there was apparently no clear demarcation in the early years between recruitment for work as a general servant and that of a nurse'. The Retreat was founded in response to the suspicious death of a Quaker patient at the subscription-based York Asylum and practised the emerging philosophy of moral management. Exemplified by the French Physician, Philippe Pinel (1745–1826), who in the 1790s allegedly freed Paris's incarcerated insane from their chains, this approach rejected the fear and force that had previously characterized treatment and promoted techniques that appealed to the patient's unimpaired faculties.[50] Therefore, although valued for their physical strength, the 'risk of personal injury' to attendants was '*very small indeed*'. In charge of between seven and ten patients, they were expected 'to clean their rooms and attend to the cleanliness of their persons'. But what the 'business of an attendant' required above all was 'a good deal of self-command and patience'.[51]

Matrons and the Voluntary Hospital

At voluntary hospitals for the physically ill, personal qualities likewise defined the role of nursing staff. Up to 1830, however, these institutions exhibited early signs of professionalization that were not apparent in asylum nursing. In common with the asylums, voluntary hospitals were either funded by a single benefactor or, more usually, by a collectivity of governors whose donations and subscriptions bought them the right to sponsor patients, participate in the general courts and weekly committees that managed the institution and elect key staff. Physicians and surgeons offered their services free of charge.[52] Both they and all the lay governors were men; and although some hospitals did form committees of 'ladies', women were not directly involved in eighteenth-century hospital management. St Bartholomew's and St Thomas' – both medieval foundations – adapted these principles to their own circumstances, but Britain's first 'true' voluntary hospital was the Westminster in London, which opened in 1720. Nursing, along with 'cleanly lodgings' and a 'wholesome diet', was regarded as integral to the delivery of care, 'found by experience to be oftentimes as effectual, towards . . . recovery . . . , as the medicines themselves'.[53] And during the course of the long eighteenth century, the matron played a managerial role in developing nursing in line with this ideal.

Hospital matrons were placed in a gendered relationship with the resident apothecary, modelled on the paternalistic domestic household. Accordingly, the apothecary was the dominant partner with wages that reflected his superiority. In 1770, for example, the *Rules* of the new Radcliffe Infirmary at Oxford set out a basic salary of £50 per annum for the apothecary, compared with only £15 for the matron.[54] Despite this pay differential, the matron's position conferred social prestige as the senior female member of staff and the governors sought suitably 'sober and discreet' recruits[55] from respectable backgrounds, often attracting the daughters or widows of clergymen, tradesmen or other men from the professional or commercial middling sort, who were drawn by the requirement to be resident. The subjection of the matron to the same electoral process as the medical staff acknowledged the importance of her role. Jacques Carré has argued that she concentrated on domestic management while the apothecary handled medical treatment.[56] This polarization is too simplistic. Despite being medically qualified via apprenticeship, apothecaries were of lower professional status than physicians or surgeons, and when employed by voluntary hospitals were expected to assume administrative as well as medical tasks.[57] Conversely, the matron's wide-ranging responsibilities were more than domestic.

Though the details varied from hospital to hospital, the matron's principal duties were threefold: the supervision of staff; the management of patients; and the procurement of provisions, furniture and household goods. First, matrons had a broad brief to supervise staff. As the matron of London's St Bartholomew's Hospital recognized in 1771, 'the happiness and quiet of the patients greatly depends upon the qualification and disposition of the persons employed to attend them'. Therefore, much of her time was spent 'enquiring after their characters, interposing in ... disputes and squabbles between the sisters, nurses, helpers and patients, and removing the sisters and nurses into different wards as their capacities best suit'.[58] Misbehaviour was taken seriously. When the authority of the matron and the apothecary was challenged by male and female servants at the Devon and Exeter Infirmary in 1774, the general court was quick to summon the culprits and instruct them to obey orders 'as you would those of your masters and mistresses in a private family'; any further misconduct would lead to discharge 'with disgrace'.[59]

The matron's second task of managing patients began with their arrival at the hospital. Since access to treatment normally required the sponsorship of a governor, she was only allowed to authorize the admission of accident or emergency cases. At some institutions, however, she did receive female patients approved by the governing body, take custody of their possessions, allocate their beds and attend the weekly meeting of physicians, surgeons and governors at which discharges were discussed.[60] Furthermore, as a senior resident member of staff, the matron regulated the behaviour of all patients. Therefore, when she reported drunkenness or smoking, abusive language or violent behaviour, damaging hospital property or being absent without leave, the governors endorsed her complaints without equivocation, expelling, reprimanding or denying the offender future recourse to a hospital bed.[61] Her role in the determination of medical treatment was more contained. In 1774, for example, both the matron and the apothecary at the Newcastle Infirmary were instructed not to move patients from one ward to another without the consent of a physician or surgeon after a dispute about the admission of infectious fever cases.[62] Furthermore, the matron of the Middlesex Hospital was suspended in 1747 when she became embroiled in a dispute between two physicians about how many maternity beds to allocate in response to the growing popularity of man-midwifery.[63]

The matron's third task was the procurement of provisions, furniture and household goods. Purchasing incidental items such as clothes for patients, bedding, table cloths and curtains normally required the authorization of the governors.[64] So too did any improvement to the physical fabric. Thus when the matron of the Newcastle Infirmary 'desired' a larger window in the wash-house, the weekly committee agreed to her request and then instructed her to make the necessary arrangements.[65] With basic foodstuffs, the matron occasionally engaged in one-off purchases as at Exeter during the 1740s when she bought cider with the apothecary and cheese and soap with a governor at the Lammas Fair.[66] For the most part, however, such items were obtained through a system of competitive tendering.[67] Whatever the method of acquisition, quality was not guaranteed and when patients at Exeter complained about the meat during the weekly committee's 1765 visitation, the matron was 'called in' and 'directed to acquaint the butcher ... [with the problem] and order him to be more careful for the future to keep up to his contract'.[68]

The quantity as well as the quality of food consumed was an issue. Although dietary tables drawn up by the physicians and surgeons determined what patients ate, financial accounts were not always accepted without question. In 1775, for example, the matron of the Radcliffe Infirmary was reminded to 'strictly adhere to the diet table' and make sure that 'all articles under her department ... [were] delivered out by weight and measure'.[69] Yet there were times when flexibility was conferred. Between 1793 and 1815, the inflationary effects of the Napoleonic Wars put voluntary hospitals under enormous pressure, particularly because grain prices fluctuated wildly and pushed up the price of bread.[70] Cutbacks had to be made.[71] However, when patients at the Newcastle Infirmary complained about how much bread they received, the matron was given 'a discretionary power to distribute ... [it] to those patients that require ... over and above the usual allowance'. In response to fuel economies, the 'old woman' wanting fire at night was permitted 'to go into the kitchen to warm herself'.[72]

The matron's tour of inspection – once or sometimes twice a day – was a common device for ensuring that she fulfilled her three functions of supervising staff, managing patients and overseeing supplies.[73] Of course, if she herself was incompetent or corrupt – like the matron of the Manchester Infirmary[74] sacked in 1808 for embezzlement – this aspiration was frustrated. But such incidents were relatively isolated. Therefore, it is surprising that the detailed knowledge of matrons was not exploited by appointing them *ex officio* members of the general courts and weekly committees that ran voluntary hospitals, or by co-opting them to serve on the *ad hoc* sub-committees set up to investigate matters that were central to their role.[75] As it was, matrons communicated their views in two ways: first, through the (male) house visitors nominated by the committee to inspect the hospital on a regular basis; and, second, in the book where these house visitors both recorded their own findings and read the requests and complaints that staff entered.[76]

House visiting was a defective mechanism for representing the matron in hospital management. To begin with, there were difficulties in sustaining a frequent flow of visitors once the enthusiasm generated by new foundations waned.[77] Moreover, even when the system was operating effectively, there was no direct access to the governors. That matrons were held in great regard was demonstrated by the pensions that they received on retirement; Mrs Whybrow was granted an annuity of £60 for life when she left Addenbrooke's Hospital, Cambridge, in 1834, 'on account of the length of her service and the exemplary manner in which ... she has invariably discharged the duties of her office'.[78] Yet despite this esteem, the matron remained bound to the rules that attached to her post, which were hung on her office walls[79] or read to her at the general court approving her appointment.[80] Therefore, we have to qualify Baly and Skeet's judgement that the status of the matron was high relative to the position of her counterparts in the twentieth-century municipal infirmaries where doctors acted as intermediaries between nursing and the management board.[81]

Nurses and the Voluntary Hospital

The hospital nurses, whose oversight formed part of the matron's job description, were not a monolithic category. St Bartholomew's and St Thomas' in London both retained the title 'sister' from the pre-Reformation period and this term was also adopted by Guy's Hospital when it opened in 1724. Although these sisters ran wards and supervised day nurses, night nurses and other assistants, they also performed tasks 'very similar to those of nurses in other infirmaries'.[82] Listed as servants in hospital rule books, nurses were instructed to 'obey the Matron as their Mistress' and to clean their wards by a specified time each morning. 'Tenderness' towards patients was also required, together with 'Civility and Respect' towards 'Strangers' or visitors.[83] In return for their efforts, hospital nurses earned significantly more than hospital servants. Therefore, when Hannah Harris was appointed as a nurse at the Exeter Infirmary in 1743, her wages were £5 per annum: almost double the £2 15 shillings paid to Martha Warren as a housemaid.[84] In addition to a salary, nurses received board and lodgings. Both terms and conditions were taken seriously. When the Radcliffe Infirmary hired a night nurse in 1830, her pay was augmented after she mistakenly supposed that tea and sugar were available as a perquisite.[85] Four years before, the Infirmary had increased wages and gratuities following a petition from nurses, although the discretionary awards were dependent upon a recommendation of good conduct from the medical staff.[86]

Poor remuneration, with wages comparable to those of a domestic servant, has been blamed for the recruitment of nurses 'from the lowest rungs of society without any special knowledge or commitment to the job'.[87] Carol Helmstadter has shown that the nineteenth-century London teaching hospitals did have difficulty in employing suitable nurses.[88] However, it cannot be assumed that eighteenth-century nurses were equally drunken and profligate, especially at the provincial infirmaries. Before 1800 there were undoubtedly incidences of misbehaviour. Nurses neglected patients, they stole money from them, they misappropriated hospital property, they indulged in alcohol, they quarrelled with each other, they were rude to fellow staff and they went absent without leave. Indeed, Alice McCann, a nurse at Mercer's Hospital, Dublin, was in 1738 'carried before the Lord Mayor to be punished for seducing the Patients in the House'.[89] Nevertheless, it is important to keep these transgressions in perspective. For at the Bath Infirmary the minutes record that between 1742 and 1830 only 19 nurses were dismissed for misconduct: hardly indicative of a breakdown of order.[90] Therefore, it is important to avoid the historiographical rupture imposed by nineteenth-century reformers to strengthen the case for change and acknowledge the deeper roots of professionalization in the Georgian era.

The eighteenth century was a critical period for the professions as lawyers, clergy and medical men sought to consolidate their wealth, status and power.[91] In nursing, of course, there was no such sharp trajectory. However, we do see traces of the agenda for moral reform that animated the nursing sisterhoods from the 1830s and signs of the expertise in bodily and clinical care that had become essential to medical practice by 1900. Moral reform was integral to the mission of the voluntary hospital, which sought to 'improve' patients at a time when disease and injury dismantled resistance to change.[92] The regulatory codes designed for this purpose were applied also to nurses, so both groups were forbidden to consume alcohol, swear, behave indecently, smoke or play at dice and cards.[93] But having common rules put nurses in an 'uneasy position' because – unlike the governors, physicians and surgeons, apothecary and matron – they were present in the wards on a regular basis and hence at the coalface of patient discipline. Over time their role evolved as they began to take an active part in upholding the regulations and reporting misdemeanours. Therefore, William Cullen, physician to the Edinburgh Infirmary, used nurses to guard against malingering. Lecturing to medical students in 1772, he disclosed that he had 'employed the nurse to let me know whether the patient made me a fair report'.[94]

As well as policing their charges, nurses were increasingly expected to be 'living examples of virtue and prudence'.[95] The Evangelical Revival, which swept through the Protestant churches from the 1730s, equated respectability with literacy as well as emphasized salvation by faith. Therefore, we can interpret the imposition of reading tests from the 1780s as a bid for this more moral nurse.[96] However, literacy also supported the expertise that nursing was beginning to accumulate. The aperture was the requirement to be tender to patients, which evinced the 'aspiration to create a caring environment'.[97] Before 1830, domestic tasks were undertaken by servants *and* nurses, and hospital rules demanded that patients who were able not only wash, iron and clean the wards but also nurse other patients:[98] a duty not officially asked of nurses. Yet despite these confused boundaries, a distinctive nursing role was slowly emerging to encompass both the bodily and the clinical needs of patients.

Attention to *bodily* needs resulted from a more detailed specification of what nurses should do. In 1788 – sandwiched between advice on how frequently sheets were to be changed, and floors and chamber pots scoured – the matron of the Manchester Infirmary was thus allowed extra nurses 'so that the legs and arms of every patient could be washed with soap and water after admission, and that such washing be often repeated unless ordered to the contrary'.[99] Attention to *clinical* needs was evident from the foundation of voluntary hospitals. In 1752, for example, nurses at the Newcastle Infirmary were instructed 'to see that all the in-patients take their medicines' after a patient had destroyed her prescription.[100] By the early nineteenth century, physicians and surgeons were seeking a greater nursing input and when the medical committee at the General Hospital in Birmingham complained that 'nurses were absent from the wards for long periods of time because they were occupied in washing', the matron was told 'to find alternative labour for this task'.[101]

The interest in nursing was indicative of evolving medical knowledge and practice. Though medical knowledge was dominated by the humoral system, mechanical and chemical theories were grafted on to this basic model, and by the late eighteenth century it was being displaced by a localized pathology that focused on discrete body organs.[102] For voluntary hospitals committed to the advance of medical practice,[103] these changes had significant effects, and from an early stage machines were purchased and operating theatres were opened with adjoining wards for post-operative patients.[104] Nurses were not invariably affected. At Manchester in 1791, for instance, a man and a woman – not nurses – were recruited to attend patients after operations and to provide surgeons with 'proper dressings and bandages' both in the wards and for emergency admissions.[105] Over time, however, as medicine embraced an increasingly scientific methodology, hospital physicians and surgeons required an ancillary staff with sufficient clinical expertise to follow more complex instructions and to report pertinent alterations in the patient's condition.[106] It was nurses who were expected to assume these new responsibilities and doctors complained when they fell short. At Edinburgh, Cullen grumbled in his lectures that the feet of a rheumatic patient 'were allowed to be cold and the sweat did not continue half of the time owing to the negligence of the nurse or her want of skill'.[107] At the Radcliffe Infirmary, Nurse Stanbridge was sacked in 1806 'for the neglect of Mrs Wilsden after the operation of couching' to treat a cataract.[108]

The solidity of the pre-reform nursing role should not be exaggerated because hospitals continued to aggregate nursing and domestic work.[109] However, there was enough movement towards patients' bodily and clinical needs to suggest that a nascent professionalization was underway. Patients' responses to this nursing care are largely missing, but in 1809 an actor called Joseph Wilde penned a long poem describing his nine-week stay at the Exeter Hospital. Fulsome in his praise of the institution, the physicians and the patient community, Wilde exhibits a 'virulent antipathy to the nursing staff', 'ungracious and unfeeling women who for him are the veritable embodiment of uncharitable behaviour':[110] 'such the cruel nature of this pest', he wrote, 'Her tongue kills more than ablest doctors cure.'[111] This evaluation is qualified if not overturned by the generosity that hospitals showed towards their nurses. At Exeter itself the weekly committee ordered in 1758 that 'leave be given to Nurse Batten and Nurse Hoard to go into the country for the benefit of the air'.[112] Pensions were also granted in return for loyal service and good conduct. Therefore, when she became 'infirm' at the age of 68 in 1793, Nurse Catherine Green was awarded 'the sum of four shillings weekly' on the grounds that she 'behaved in every respect to the satisfaction of the governors' during her 20 years' service to the Radcliffe Infirmary.[113]

Conclusion

Nurses between 1700 and 1830 were a miscellaneous group with loci of care in family households, the local community, military institutions, workhouses, asylums and hospitals. The issues of ethnicity that were to affect the twentieth-century profession were far distant. Social class too was still to bite. Paid nurses were generally drawn from the lower orders but these labouring classes had yet to forge a strong class identity built around economic, social, political and cultural power.[114] At least some matrons inhabited a more ambivalent position on the margins of a middling sort that by the late eighteenth century was beginning to mature into a middle class.[115] Occupationally, however, they were subordinate to the apothecary, who himself sat below physicians and surgeons in the medical hierarchy. Gender as well as status underwrote this inter-professional relationship, as in all contexts the association of nursing with women was consolidated. Nevertheless, the recognition of non-child nursing as an activity in its own right, the employment of nurses by the Poor Law and charitable bodies and − critically − the embryonic concern for the bodily and clinical needs of voluntary hospital patients prefigure the professionalization that was to gather momentum in the nineteenth century. Therefore, we have to reject Brian Abel-Smith's contention that in 1800 'nursing amounted to little more than a specialized form of charring'.[116]

Acknowledgements

I am grateful to staff at the Devon Record Office, the Oxfordshire Health Archives and the Tyne and Wear Archives for their help with the archival aspects of this chapter.

Notes

1. C. Dickens, *The Life and Adventures of Martin* Chuzzlewit, 1st pub. in serial form in 1843 and as a novel in 1844 (London: Oxford University Press, 1951) p. 313.
2. A. Summers, 'The Mysterious Demise of Sarah Gamp: The Domiciliary Nurse and Her Detractors, *c.*1830−1860', *Victorian Studies*, 32:3 (1989) 365.
3. C. Rawcliffe, 'Hospital Nurses and Their Work', in R. Britnell (ed.), *Daily Life in the Middle Ages* (Stroud: Alan Sutton, 1998) pp. 53−4; L. McCray Beier, 'In Sickness and in Health: A Seventeenth Century Family's Experience', in R. Porter (ed.), *Patients and Practitioners: Lay Perceptions of Medicine in Pre-Industrial Society* (Cambridge: Cambridge University Press, 1985) pp. 102−28.
4. M. Pelling and C. Webster, 'Medical Practitioners', in C. Webster (ed.), *Health, Medicine and Mortality in the Sixteenth Century* (Cambridge: Cambridge University Press, 1979) p. 166.
5. K. Thomas, *Religion and the Decline of Magic: Studies in Popular Beliefs in Sixteenth- and Seventeenth-Century England*, 1st pub. 1971 (Harmondsworth: Penguin, 1973) pp. 11−15; M. Baly, *Nursing and Social Change*, 1st pub. 1973, 3rd edn (London: Routledge, 1995) pp. 41−2.

6. G. Smith, 'Prescribing the Rules of Health: Self-Help and Advice in the Late Eighteenth Century', in Porter (ed.), *Patients and Practitioners*, p. 280.

7. R. Porter, *The Greatest Benefit to Mankind: A Medical History of Humanity from Antiquity to the Present* (London: HarperCollins, 1997) pp. 55–62.

8. S. King, *A Fylde Country Practice: Medicine and Society in Lancashire, c.1760–1840* (Lancaster: Centre for North-West Regional Studies, 2001) pp. 44–5, 57.

9. W. Cadogan, *An Essay upon the Nursing and Management of Children, from Their Birth to Three Years of Age*, 2nd edn (London: J. Roberts, 1748).

10. H. Smith, *Letter to Married Women on Nursing and the Management of Their Children*, 6th edn (London: C. and G. Kearsley, 1792). Although the sixth edition was published in 1792, the text is dated 1774.

11. Smith, *Letter*, pp. iii–iv, ix.

12. Smith, *Letter*, pp. 199–202, 213, 217–22.

13. K. Gleadle, *British Women in the Nineteenth Century* (Basingstoke: Palgrave Macmillan, 2001) pp. 4–5.

14. D. Gibson (ed.), *A Parson in the Vale of White Horse: George Woodward's Letters from East Hendred, 1753–1761* (Stroud: Alan Sutton, 1982) p. 129.

15. T. Sokoll, 'Old Age in Poverty: The Record of Essex Pauper Letters, 1780–1834', in T. Hitchcock, P. King and P. Sharp (eds), *Chronicling Poverty: The Voices and Strategies of the English Poor, 1640–1840* (Basingstoke: Macmillan, 1997) p. 136.

16. King, *A Fylde Country Practice*, p. 37.

17. A. Withey, 'Medicine, Healing and the Family in Wales, 1600–1750', Swansea University, PhD thesis (2009) p. 262.

18. C. Elmsley, T. Hitchcock and R. Shoemaker, 'Publishing History of the Proceedings from Their Inception in 1764 to the Final Issue in 1913', *Old Bailey Proceedings Online* [*OBP*] (www.oldbaileyonline.org), 20 February 2010; C. Elmsley, T. Hitchcock and R. Shoemaker, 'The Value of the Proceedings as a Historical Source', *OBP*, 20 February 2010.

19. *OBP*, 19 February 2010, February 1795, trial of Deborah Sheene (t17950218-25). All subsequent references to the *OBP* were accessed on the same date.

20. *OBP*, January 1798, trial of John Wheeler, Thomas Hall (t17980110-40).

21. *OBP*, September 1752, trial of Ann Edwards, Benjamin Edwards, Mary Edwards, Millicent Edwards (t17520914-40).

22. *OBP*, December 1828, trial of Elizabeth Davies (t18281204-103).

23. *OBP*, May 1799, trial of Francis Chant (t17990508-49).

24. *OBP*, July 1730, trial of Alice Leader (t17300704-36); *OBP*, April 1743, trial of Elizabeth Stuart (t17430413-51).
25. *OBP*, January 1748, trial of Isaac Fletcher (t17480115-7); *OBP*, September 1788, trial of Martha Daniels (t17880910-28).
26. *OBP*, February 1796, trial of John Martin (t17960217-21).
27. *OBP*, May 1826, trial of Hannah Green (t18260511-4).
28. *OBP*, April 1750, trial of William Archer (t17500425-24).
29. S. Williams, 'Caring for the Sick Poor', in P. Lane, N. Raven and K.D.M. Snell (eds), *Women, Work and Wages in England, 1600–1850* (Woodbridge: Boydell, 2004) pp. 149–51, 162–5.
30. A. Brundage, *The English Poor Laws, 1700–1930* (Basingstoke: Palgrave Macmillan, 2002) pp. 25, 39.
31. *OBP*, October 1761, trial of Richard Parrott (t17611021-34).
32. M.D. George, *London Life in the Eighteenth Century*, 1st pub. 1925 (Harmondsworth: Penguin, 1966) pp. 68, 215, 371.
33. R. McClure, *Coram's Children: The London Foundling Hospital in the Eighteenth Century* (New Haven: Yale University Press, 1981) pp. 37, 87–92, 94.
34. George, *London Life*, p. 17.
35. *OBP*, April 1798, trial of Margaret Bladon (t17980418-109).
36. *OBP*, December 1731, trial of Elizabeth Smith (t17311208-13); *OBP*, September 1788, trial of Martha Daniels (t17880910-28); *OBP*, July 1814, trial of Harriot Marks (t18140706-17).
37. *OBP*, December 1741, trial of Christopher Shotton (t17411204-28).
38. *OBP*, December 1744, trial of Ann Collier (t17441205-61).
39. *OBP*, November 1794, trial of Susannah Milesent (017941111-1); *OBP*, October 1826, trial of Henry Cleaveland (t18261026-251).
40. *OBP*, October 1801, trial of James Legg (t18011028-39).
41. J. Dobson, 'The Army Nursing Service in the Eighteenth Century', *Annals of the Royal College of Surgeons*, 14 (1954) 417–19.
42. J. Boulton, 'Welfare Systems and the Parish Nurse in Early Modern London, 1650–1725', *Family and Community History*, 10:2 (2007) 147–8.
43. P. Slack, *The English Poor Law, 1531–1782* (Basingstoke: Macmillan, 1990) pp. 39–45.
44. R. White, *Social Change and the Development of the Nursing Profession: A Study of the Poor Law Nursing Service, 1848–1948* (London: Henry Kimpton, 1978) pp. 5–6.
45. *OBP*, January 1757, trial of Martha Perry (t17570114-24); *OBP*, April 1805, trial of Martha Hunt (t18050424-93); *OBP*, April 1809, trial of Sarah Liddle (t18090412-64).
46. *OBP*, September 1812, trial of Ann Hudson (t18120916-170).
47. *OBP*, December 1732, trial of Richard Albridge (t17321206-5).

48. R. Porter, *Mind-Forg'd Manacles: A History of Madness in England from the Restoration to the Regency*, 1st pub. 1987 (London: Penguin, 1990) pp. 122, 130–4, 164–5.
49. J. Andrews, A. Briggs, R. Porter, P. Tucker and K. Waddington, *The History of Bethlem* (London: Routledge, 1997) pp. 273, 290, 292, 297.
50. R. Porter, *Mind-Forg'd Manacles: A History of Madness in England from the Restoration to the Regency* (London: Penguin, 1987) p. 6.
51. A. Digby, *Madness, Morality and Medicine: A Study of the York Retreat, 1796–1914* (Cambridge: Cambridge University Press, 1985) pp. 12, 34, 142, 144, 153–4.
52. R. Porter, 'The Gift Relation: Philanthropy and Provincial Hospitals in Eighteenth-Century England', in L. Granshaw and R. Porter (eds), *The Hospital in History* (London: Routledge, 1989) pp. 149–78.
53. *An Account of the Proceedings of the Charitable Society for Relieving the Sick and Needy at the Publick Infirmary in Westminster* (London: no publisher, 1733) p. 4.
54. *Rules and Orders for the Government of the Radcliffe Infirmary* (Oxford: W. Jackson, 1770) pp. 15–16.
55. *An Account of the Rise, Progress, and State of the London Infirmary ...'* (London: no publisher, 1742) p. 4.
56. J. Carré, 'Hospital Nurses in Eighteenth-Century Britain: Service without Responsibility', in I. Baudino, J. Carré and Cécile Révauger (eds), *The Invisible Woman: Aspects of Women's Work in Eighteenth-Century Britain* (Aldershot: Ashgate, 2005) pp. 92–3.
57. J. Woodward, *To Do the Sick No Harm: A Study of the British Voluntary Hospital System to 1875* (London: Routledge and Kegan Paul, 1974) pp. 28–9.
58. G. Yeo, *Nursing at Bart's: A History of Nurse Service and Nurse Education at St Bartholomew's Hospital, London* (Stroud: Alan Sutton, 1995) pp. 13–14.
59. Devon Record Office [DRO], Devon and Exeter Hospital, 1260 F/HM2, General Court Book, Vol. II, 25 January 1774.
60. DRO, 1260 F/HS 1, *Statutes and Constitutions of the Devon and Exeter Hospital at Exeter*, Twelve Tables of Rules and Orders for the Government and Conduct of the House, pp. 19, 24.
61. Tyne and Wear Archives [TWA], Royal Victoria Hospital, HO. RV1/2/1, House Committee Minutes, 5 August 1753; HO. RV1/2/6, House Committee Minutes, 20 July 1769; HO. RV1/2/11, House Committee Minutes, 10 October 1798.
62. TWA, HO. RVI/2/6, House Committee Minutes, 20 January 1774, 27 January 1774, 3 February 1774.
63. M. Baly and M. Skeet, *A History of Nursing at the Middlesex Hospital, 1945–1990* (London: Middlesex Hospital Nurses' Benevolent Fund, 2000) p. 3.

64. DRO, 1260 F/HM13, Committee of Governors, 5 December 1765, 4 September 1766; TWA, HO. RV1/2/1, House Committee Minutes, 30 May 1751; Oxfordshire Health Archives [OHA], Radcliffe Infirmary, RI C 1/1, Weekly Board, 24 October 1776; RI 1 C 1/3, Weekly Board, 10 April 1799.
65. TWA, HO. RVI/2/1, House Committee Minutes, 1 August 1751.
66. DRO, 1260 F/HM8, Committee of Governors, 26 July 1744, 7 November 1745.
67. A. Borsay, *Medicine and Charity in Georgian Bath: A Social History of the General Infirmary, c.1739–1830* (Aldershot: Ashgate, 1999) pp. 38–9.
68. DRO, 1260 F/HM13, Committee of Governors, 25 July 1765.
69. OHA, RI 1 C 1/1, Weekly Board, 7 March 1775.
70. E.J. Evans, *The Forging of the Modern State: Early Industrial Britain, 1783–1870* (London: Longman, 1983) pp. 81–5.
71. H. Saunders, *The Middlesex Hospital, 1745–1948* (London: Max Parrish, 1949) p. 18.
72. TWA, HO. RV1/2/11, House Committee Minutes, 29 August 1799, 3 October 1799.
73. *Laws, Orders and Regulations of the Middlesex Hospital for Sick and Lame Patients, Lying-In Married Women, and Persons Afflicted with Cancer* (London: J. Smeeton, 1793) p. 33.
74. W. Brockbank, *The History of Nursing at the M.R.I., 1752–1929* (Manchester: Manchester University Press, 1970) p. 18.
75. TWA, HO. RV1/2/1, House Committee Minutes, 20 September 1753; DRO, 1260F/HM2, General Court Book, Vol. II, 1 December 1768.
76. *Laws of the London Infirmary* (London: H. Woodfall, 1743) p. 8.
77. TWA, HO. RV1/72/5, *A Report of the State of the Infirmary for the Sick and Lame Poor of the Counties of Durham, Newcastle Upon Tyne, and Northumberland, for the 30th Year, ending April 4th, 1781.*
78. A. Rook, M. Carlton and W.G. Cannon, *The History of Addenbrooke's Hospital, Cambridge* (Cambridge: Cambridge University Press, 1991) p. 88.
79. Brockbank, *History*, p. 12.
80. DRO, 1260 F/HM 2, General Court Book, Vol. II, 25 January 1763.
81. Baly and Skeet, *History*, pp. 5–6.
82. Carré, 'Hospital Nurses', p. 91.
83. *Rules and Orders of the Public Infirmary at Liverpool* (Liverpool: J. Sadler, 1749) p. 23.
84. DRO, 1260 F/HM 8, Committee of Governors, 27 May 1743, 22 September 1743.
85. OHA, RI 1 C /7, Weekly Board, 27 January 1830.
86. OHA, RI 1 C /6, Weekly Board, 26 October 1826.

87. P. Williams, 'Religion, Respectability and the Origins of the Modern Nurse', in R. French and A. Wear (eds), *British Medicine in an Age of Reform* (London: Routledge, 1991) p. 233.
88. C. Helmstadter, 'Nurse Recruitment and Retention in the Nineteenth-Century London Teaching Hospitals', *International History of Nursing Journal* 2:1 (1996) 58, 61–2.
89. J.B. Lyons, *The Quality of Mercer's: The Story of Mercer's Hospital, 1735–1991* (Dublin: Glendale, 1991).
90. Borsay, *Medicine*, pp. 353–4.
91. P.J. Corfield, *Power and the Professions in Britain, 1700–1850* (London: Routledge, 1995).
92. *An Address to the Nobility, Gentry, Clergy, and Others on Behalf of a Public Infirmary Now Erected at Liverpool*, in G. McLoughlin (eds), *A Short History of the First Liverpool Infirmary, 1749–1824* (Chichester: Phillimore, 1978) p. 17.
93. J. Wood, *A Description of Bath 1765* (Bath: Kingsmead Reprints, 1969) pp. 295, 297–9.
94. G.B. Risse, *Hospital Life in Enlightenment Scotland: Care and Teaching at the Royal Infirmary of Edinburgh* (Cambridge: Cambridge University Press, 1986) p. 78.
95. Carré, 'Hospital Nurses', pp. 98–9.
96. R. Dingwall, A.-M. Rafferty and C. Webster, *An Introduction to the Social History of Nursing* (London: Routledge, 1998) p. 19.
97. Dingwall, Rafferty and Webster, *Social History*, p. 11.
98. *Rules and Orders of the Public Infirmary at Liverpool*, p. 24.
99. Brockbank, *History*, pp. 9–11.
100. TWA, HO. RV1/2/1, House Committee Minutes, 27 February 1752.
101. S. Wildman, 'The Development of Nursing at the General Hospital, Birmingham, 1779–1919', *International History of Nursing Journal*, 4:3 (1999) 21.
102. N.D. Jewson, 'Medical Knowledge and the Patronage System in Eighteenth Century England', *Sociology*, VIII (1974) 371–2.
103. 'A View of the Many Peculiar Advantages of Publick Hospitals', *Gentleman's Magazine*, XI (1741) 746–7.
104. See, for example, DRO, 1260 F/HM 11, Committee of Governors, 13 May 1756; DRO, 1260 F/HM 13, Committee of Governors, 6 November 1766, 21 July 1768; DRO, 1260 F/HM 17, Committee of Governors, 13 April 1795.
105. Brockbank, *History*, p. 11.
106. Dingwall, Rafferty and Webster, *Social History*, pp. 22–3.
107. Risse, *Hospital Life*, p. 78.
108. OHA, RI 1 C /4, Weekly Board, 10 July 1806.
109. OHA, RI 1 C /5, Weekly Board, 20 January 1820.

110. R. Porter, 'The Gift Relation', in L. Granshaw and R. Porter (eds), *The Hospital in History* (London: Routledge, 1989) pp. 169–72.
111. J. Wilde, *The Hospital*, cited in W.B. Howie, 'Consumer Reaction: A Patient's View of Hospital Life in 1809', *British Medical Journal*, 3 (1973) 536.
112. DRO, 1260 F/HM 11, Committee of Governors, 15 November 1758.
113. OHA, RI 1 C /3, Weekly Board, 2 October 1793.
114. J. Rule, *Albion's People: English Society, 1714–1815* (London: Longman, 1992) pp. 105–8.
115. Borsay, *Medicine*, pp. 386–7.
116. B. Abel-Smith, *A History of the Nursing Profession* (London: Heinemann, 1960) p. 4.

3

Nursing, 1830–1920: Forging a Profession

Christine E. Hallett

The view that nursing was forged as a profession during the nineteenth century is widely held and largely unchallenged. The period was indeed one of significant change in which nursing acquired professional status, prestige and material gain for its members.[1] It would be impossible to explore every aspect of these developments. Instead, this chapter will focus primarily on general nursing between 1830 and 1920: the years in which the most dramatic changes took place.

The 'Pre-Reform' Nurse

Despite the best efforts of historians to play down the importance of Charles Dickens's fictional character, Sarah Gamp, the nursing profession cannot escape her legacy. Nor does it seem to wish to. From the 1850s onwards, those who deliberately promoted the development of nursing as a 'new' and 'reformed' discipline drew very deliberately on the images of Gamp and her colleague, Betsy Prig, to accentuate both the extent to which nursing had redeemed itself, and the dangers that were posed by any backsliding into the old ways.

The nature of the 'pre-reform' nurse has been the subject of much debate. No doubt some truly were Gamps – uneducated, surly, disinterested characters who reeked of gin and snuff. Others, as Barbara Mortimer has persuasively shown, in the context of mid-nineteenth-century Edinburgh, were hardworking women of society's lower orders who acquired experience and expertise over the course of long and successful independent careers. Mortimer used Post Office directories for 1834–1871 and the Census enumerator's books for 1861 to trace the lives and work of these 'shadowy' and 'elusive creatures'. She argues that the private nurses of Edinburgh were not seen as part of a wider group of domestic servants. Their work was, rather, placed alongside other commercial enterprises, such as millinery and dressmaking. Those who listed themselves as 'sick nurse', or 'lady's nurse' (some of whom were also 'midwives'), may have been some of the most successful small businesswomen of the nineteenth century.[2] Anne Summers had earlier argued that many of those Londoners who appear in the 1861 Census as 'nurse, not domestic servant' were probably independent practitioners working, perhaps, in direct competition with doctors offering long-term care to those with minor ailments, injuries and chronic illnesses and who could afford to pay for their services.[3]

Hospital care has also been subject to the mythologizing treatment of mid-century reformers.[4] For London if not the provinces, there may be some truth in accounts that some nurses subjected their patients to rough handling and cruel treatment; that the taking of bribes was routine in some hospitals; and that the condition of the nurses themselves was much to be pitied due to long hours of arduous menial work, little pay beyond their keep and accommodation, often, in attics, tiny cells or even 'cages' on the landings outside their hospital wards.[5] Conditions were worst in Poor Law institutions, which became the subject of campaigns by visitors like Louisa Twining whose writings laid the foundations for the subsequent philanthropic efforts of nurse-reformers.[6] Ann Simnett has studied one Poor Law Hospital, belonging to the Billericay Union in South East Essex. Here, even by the 1860s, 'although the wages of the paid nurses in the workhouse infirmaries were on a par with the lowliest of domestic servants, their duties as set out by the Poor Law Board were comparable with those of sisters in the London hospitals'.[7]

Mid-century nursing roles were highly gendered. Very few male nurses worked in general nursing, though large numbers could be found in asylums. The physical strength that enabled a male asylum attendant to control an aggressive patient was viewed as an important qualification in an era of restraint, before the advent of drugs and therapies designed to control violent behaviour.[8] The other realm in which large numbers of men were to be found was in the military medical services, where orderlies worked alongside medical officers under the authority of their own officers.[9] This gendering of nursing as 'women's work' has had an important impact on the status of the nursing profession. While nurses themselves saw femininity as their strength – the quality that permitted them to exercise authority in the 'domestic sphere' of the hospital ward, and to excel in both the caring and the managerial aspects of nursing work – doctors 'used the language of femininity to restrict the expansion of nursing'.[10]

The Rise of Sisterhoods

The earliest moves to reform nursing coincided both with a powerful upsurge in religious and spiritual consciousness and with women's need to find an outlet from the stultification of domestic life. Martha Vicinus has argued that the juxtaposition of these drives underlay the remarkably rapid development of religious sisterhoods in the mid-nineteenth century.[11] Primarily spiritual in motivation, communities of all religious persuasions expressed their devotion through 'good works', experiencing 'the call to serve God through work with his needy'.[12]

One of the most remarkable of these movements was Catholic in origin and inspiration. In 1838 a group of Irish Sisters of Mercy established a convent in Bermondsey, south London. The sisters became highly respected by their local community, even as they aroused the suspicion of Britain's Protestant elites who feared mass conversions to Roman Catholicism. Some of their most celebrated new members, notably Lady Barbara Eyre, were drawn from British aristocratic families. Perhaps because of the diplomatic skill of their leader, Mary Clare Moore, the sisters managed to avoid controversy and were remarkably successful, founding 22 houses in England and winning the respect of Florence Nightingale through their work in the Crimea.[13] However, their influence on the development of nursing as a practice or as a profession was limited. Of more importance were those Anglican sisterhoods that offered their services to some of the more influential London hospitals, and thereby exerted an important influence on contemporary ideas about the development of nursing.

The forerunner of the Protestant sisterhoods was the Institute for Nursing Sisters, founded in London by Elizabeth Fry in 1840.[14] The Institute took on women of good character, and offered them hands-on training on the wards of Guy's Hospital in London, to equip them to offer nursing care to the sick poor in their own homes. Fry, along with the founders of other sisterhoods, was influenced by the example of the deaconess institute established by Theodore

Fliedner and his wife, Friedericke, at Kaiserswerth in Germany.[15] English Protestantism encompassed a range of different religious persuasions, from low-church Methodism to high-church Anglicanism, and Protestant sisterhoods came to represent these different forms.[16] Anne Summers and Sioban Nelson have shown how influential the nursing sisterhoods were. St John's House, the All Saints Sisterhood, the Holy Rood and the Community of St Margaret offer particularly important case studies. All trained their nurses within, and offered their services to, influential London voluntary hospitals.[17] All consisted of an essentially two-tier system, in which genteel 'ladies' – the 'sisters' – offered discipline, training and guidance to working-class 'nurses' who gave most of the actual nursing care. Particular attention has been given to St John's House, partly because of the influence of its leader, Mary Jones, on Florence Nightingale.[18]

Judith Moore's study of St John's House provides a clear window to the tensions and conflicts that surrounded the Anglican sisterhoods. Founded as a 'Training Institution for Nurses in Hospitals, Families and for the Poor', the Order of St John the Evangelist was established in 1848 under the influence of medical reformer Robert Bentley Todd.[19] The importance of this medical influence cannot be underestimated. Todd and his contemporaries saw an increasing need for efficient, effective and humane care for hospital patients in the face of more complex scientific medicine, in which the interventions of the doctor could be potentially as dangerous as the disease itself. However, they couched this need as an essentially medical one, synonymous with the requirement that the doctor should have an effective assistant to carry out his 'orders'. This medical autocracy, along with the power of the male governing council of St John's House and the religious sectarian tensions that surrounded it, was to lead to repeated conflict and ultimately to the fracturing of the sisterhood.[20]

By the 1860s, St John's House was providing and overseeing the nursing care at King's College Hospital, Charing Cross Hospital and the Hospital for Sick Children in Nottingham. It provided a clear precedent for the model of clinical nursing that was to develop over the last four decades of the nineteenth century. The nurses of St John's House offered a 'high standard of postsurgical care' and this, along with their refusal to take on menial ward-cleaning work, created a system of nursing that was to inspire future reforms. The conflicts and tensions they experienced also taught the new reformers that any future nursing services must avoid sectarianism. The religious sisterhoods can therefore be seen as a valuable experiment which helped confirm that British nursing would take on a pious, charitable but essentially humanistic and secular form. Religious nursing had, nevertheless, acted as 'a force for reform and a doorway for respectable women to the public domain'.[21]

The Influence of Florence Nightingale

Notwithstanding the importance of the sisterhoods, it is impossible to deny the enormous influence of Florence Nightingale on the transformation of nursing from a base occupation suitable only for the lowest orders into a profession in which royal and aristocratic women took an interest. Her work and her iconic status secured greater public support than could otherwise have been achieved, and it was this support that allowed her (and others) to push through reform.[22]

Nightingale had a clear vision of what nursing should be: any work that placed the patient in the best circumstances to enable a natural process of healing to occur.[23] The story of her life and work in implementing this vision has been recited many times.[24] Lynn McDonald has exploded a number of historical myths, among them the suggestion that the system of nursing taught at St Thomas's Hospital was nothing more than 'applied housekeeping', failing to incorporate an adequate amount of clinical training or medical knowledge.[25] She suggests that teaching at St Thomas's was in keeping with contemporary medical thinking and that it had a pervasive influence, in particular through the work of the hundreds of Nightingale probationers who became matrons in prominent hospitals throughout Britain and the rest of the world.[26] At the same time, other voluntary hospitals were introducing their own schemes for training nurses. A survey conducted by former Nightingale probationer Florence Lees in 1874 demonstrated that a number of London hospitals had effective training schools. The Middlesex, University College Hospital, King's College Hospital and Charing Cross Hospital all had training programmes – the last three run by sisterhoods.[27] Much later, in the 1890s, Eva Luckes, matron of the London Hospital, established the first systematic classroom training, in the form of the first 'preliminary training school' at Tredegar House.[28]

The 'New' Nurse

The Nightingale influence, in combination with the sisterhoods, brought about a number of rapid and significant changes in nursing during the second half of the nineteenth century. Perhaps the most obvious was a transformation in the image of the nurse herself. The two now-famous sketches, published in the *Nursing Record* for December 20, 1888 – one depicting the aged, corpulent and morally destitute Gamp gazing at a gin bottle and the other the young, pure 'new nurse' sitting alongside the Christian cross – have, for obvious reasons, been dismissed as propaganda.[29] Behind the images, though, there do seem to have been a number of trends. Nurses did become younger as the century progressed; uniforms did replace their own sometimes shabby attire; and the Christian cross did replace the gin bottle as the emblem by which society recognized them.[30] Although the evidence is patchy, and caution should be exercised when applying a few small case studies to a whole population, it would appear that a number of real changes took place during the second half of the nineteenth century, and that those changes were rapid enough to constitute a revolution in nursing.

Carol Helmstadter illustrates for the London teaching hospitals the difficulty early nineteenth-century governors and doctors experienced in 'the procuring of proper persons to act as nurses'.[31] She argues that a deliberate process of 'professionalization' took place in mid-nineteenth-century London, in which the focus was on improving the moral 'tone' of the hospital ward – a process which could only be accomplished by a 'lady' from the middle or upper classes. Helmstadter sets her work in the context of a society which was deeply divided between the working and middle classes, and in which 'riotous behaviour' and alcoholism were seen as typical of the behaviour of the lower orders. She illustrates how a concerted effort on the part of middle-class nurses, some of whom were members of sisterhoods, to transform the world of the hospital into one of sobriety, propriety and high moral standards should be located within the larger project for the 'reform of manners'. In part, this project was a political one. The assumed rebelliousness of the working class was seen as a potential threat to social stability.[32] In their bid 'to establish a more orderly, systematic, and professional approach to patient care', the 'lady-nurses' of the mid-century 'tried to treat both nurses and patients with respect'.[33]

By the 1870s, there was considerable conflict between the perceptions of these 'sisters', who saw themselves as holistic carers and healers, and those of the doctors who mistakenly believed that nurses were there to act solely as their assistants – a conflict that was heightened by sectarian tensions. By this stage, however, the 'new' nursing had gained a momentum that could not be stopped. The popularity of the 'new' nurses, their recognition by society and their obvious benefits for patient care could not be denied. And yet their religious sectarianism still aroused fear and suspicion, which meant that it was still far from certain that they would gain more than a foothold in the male-medical-dominated hospital world.

The movement of women from the middle (and occasionally the upper) classes into nursing was an important precursor to the controversial changes that were taking place. Ann Simnett's research into the social class of nurse-probationers entering St Bartholomew's Hospital in the last four decades of the nineteenth century demonstrates a 'gentrification' of nursing at the hospital. She interprets these changes in the light of two influences: first, the reforming zeal of two matrons – 'Mrs Drake', appointed in 1865, and more importantly Ethel Gordon Manson, appointed in 1881 (and better known by her later, married, name of Mrs Bedford Fenwick); and, second, the dawning realization by doctors that the 'new' nurses would make better assistants than the old working-class women. Not only did they have an immeasurably better standard of education but they also constituted a 'genteel, docile and dedicated female workforce'. The first group of probationers at St Bartholomew's began their training on 1 May 1877. Many probably had to work for a living, and saw nursing as a means to 'better themselves': to move into the middle class. Simnett has shown that, as the century progressed, the tendency to recruit working women who left their previous employment (often domestic service) and entered nursing at St Bartholomew's was replaced by the increasing recruitment of young women in their mid-twenties, who had not previously held paid employment, and whose fathers were members of the professional class. There were a particularly high number of daughters of clergymen and gentleman-farmers. In 1884, the scheme at St Bartholomew's emulated the programme at Nightingale School at St Thomas's Hospital by admitting 'special' or 'paying' probationers to the school for a period of not less than three months. This permitted wealthier 'ladies' to obtain nursing experience without binding themselves into a three-year contract.[34]

As the reform of hospital nursing began to take shape in the decades after Nightingale's Crimean exploits, it was increasingly her own 'system' of nursing that was adopted by matrons in voluntary hospitals.[35] The insistence on having one female head to whom all nurses were answerable, along with the practice of moving probationers from ward to ward so that they gained experience of a number of branches of nursing care, caused increasing tension between senior nurses and hospital doctors, who had been accustomed to exercising authority over 'their' ward nurses. Nurses, on the other hand, increasingly saw themselves as practitioners of a profession and discipline that – although including the implementation of a medical regimen – was distinct from, rather than merely an adjunct to, medicine.[36]

The friction created by this issue found its clearest and most controversial expression in the Guy's Hospital dispute of 1879/80. A newly appointed matron, Miss Margaret Elizabeth Burt, implemented a series of reforms, which involved the moving of probationers between wards. Her interventions led to a controversy that played out in the national press. Burt's 'boldest public champion',[37] probationer Margaret Lonsdale, committed a heinous crime by writing a very outspoken letter to the fashionable journal *The Nineteenth Century*.[38] She was audacious enough to suggest that doctors and medical students had appreciated the old-style working-class nurses because the latter did not exercise any moral restraint over their own, sometimes unacceptable, behaviour. The new-style nurse, an intelligent, educated woman from the 'gentle' classes, was more likely to act as her patients' advocate and to prevent (often merely by her witnessing presence) riotous behaviour by medical students and experimentation by experienced doctors.[39] Lonsdale's letter resulted in a series of angry rebuttals from medical practitioners throughout Britain, but an enquiry instigated by the hospital governors, which reported in July 1880, found in favour of Miss Burt's reforms.[40] The incident reverberated through the nursing and medical professions, bringing responses from members of both.[41] It also resulted in continuing tension at Guy's Hospital, which found its expression in debates around whether one particularly unfortunate nurse, Pleasance Louisa Ingle, had committed manslaughter by making an apparently independent decision to place a consumptive patient into a cold bath.[42]

Although the idea of a wholesale takeover of nursing by the middle and upper classes has now been discredited, there is evidence to suggest that middle-class women entered the profession in large numbers. One of the earliest empirical studies of this phenomenon, Christopher Maggs's *The Origins of General Nursing*, 'traces the emergence of [the] first generation of general nurses' in England. Maggs argues that this generation appeared between 1881 and 1914 and emerged only after the work of 'pioneers' such as Mary Jones and Florence Nightingale had prepared the way for organized training. Essentially, his work reached similar conclusions to those of Simnett's smaller-scale study, arguing that nursing was seen as a means by which women could 'better themselves'. Maggs maintains that nursing was transformed during the second half of the nineteenth century by the establishment of a system of education and skills-training, to the point where, by the early twentieth century, the 'special' or 'paying' probationers were obsolete. It was no longer seen as possible to undertake a shortened training: the skill and knowledge required by a nurse, along with the self-discipline that was needed to practice effectively, were too complex.[43]

Propagandists of the late nineteenth century, such as vocal pro-registrationist Ethel Bedford Fenwick, argued that the status of nursing had shifted dramatically. From its origins as a menial occupation, nursing had risen to become a profession. The term 'profession' is – and always has been – an ambiguous one. Defining it was as difficult for nineteenth-century thinkers as it is for us today. In modern terms, professionalism is synonymous with the closure of role boundaries by means of a legally sanctioned Register. Such closure, in turn, only becomes feasible when it is possible to demonstrate both the occupational group's importance to the well-being of society and its ownership of a distinct body of knowledge. 'Profession' for the nurses of the nineteenth century meant all these things; and yet it also represented something even more difficult to define: it identified one as a particular 'type'. In the largely closed society of the nineteenth century, 'type' was a birthright, essentially associated with membership of a particular 'social class'. Class, in turn, was closely related to both wealth and education. It was possible – though unusual – for an individual to move between classes: to rise into a higher class, or to fall to a lower one. What made nursing a 'profession' in the nineteenth century was an apparently dramatic shift in its social class base, from the lower echelons of the working class to the middle and even 'upper' classes.

The Poor Law Nurse

Although the efforts to frame a 'new' nurse were concentrated in the voluntary hospital, the Poor Law nurse was not exempt from change; indeed, one of Nightingale's most significant projects was her work to reform Poor Law nursing. England's Poor Law medical wards and infirmaries were in a desperate state. Established within the workhouse, these institutions were run by a matron – often the wife of the workhouse master – who knew little of nursing work and essentially played the role of housekeeper. The principle of 'less-eligibility' which governed the Poor Law as a whole sought to ensure that the situation of paupers was worse than that of the poorest independent labourer. It meant that wards in infirmaries were impoverished places, ill-equipped, poorly governed and under-resourced.

Nursing care was largely in the hands of pauper inmates, who were unable to earn their own living and entered the workhouse because of their own destitution. These Poor Law 'nurses' were untrained, sometimes hardened by their own experiences of poverty, and all-too-often in poor health themselves.[44] A scandal erupted in London on the Christmas Eve of 1864 when *The Times* reported the case of Timothy Daly, a pauper who had died as a result of neglect in a workhouse infirmary. This and other scandals led to the setting up of the *Lancet Commission* to investigate Poor Law medical care.[45] The work of the Commission – with the acknowledged support of Nightingale – led in 1867 to the passing of the Metropolitan Poor Law Act, the first legislation to acknowledge the duty of the state to provide hospitals for the poor.[46]

By the time the Lancet Commission reported its findings, Nightingale's own plans to develop Poor Law nursing were well in train. In 1865, in collaboration with philanthropist William Rathbone, Nightingale placed one of the Nightingale School trainees, Agnes Jones, in the Liverpool Brownlow Hill Workhouse Infirmary with a team of nurses and instructions to reform nursing care within the infirmary.[47] Jones appeared to have been inspired by an evangelical religious zeal to take on this immensely challenging work. She encountered opposition from both staff and guardians.[48]

After working in the stifling, overcrowded and impoverished environment of the Liverpool Workhouse Infirmary, Agnes Jones herself contracted typhus fever and died. There has been some controversy over whether this 'experiment' in Poor Law nursing had any long-term effects. McDonald has argued that Nightingale persisted with her work at the Liverpool Workhouse Infirmary, and that she also recommended 'Nightingale nurses' to positions at a number of workhouse infirmaries within and outside London.[49] Agnes Jones herself, Nightingale memorialized in an extraordinary article, 'Una and the Lion', which related Jones's real-life deeds to myth and legend, had the intended effect of inspiring large numbers of devout women to enter nursing.[50] In the early twentieth century, the task of improving conditions within workhouse infirmaries was taken up by reformers such as Beatrice Webb, who demanded the dismantling of the entire Poor Law system and a more equitable distribution of health care.[51]

The District Nurse

Florence Nightingale believed that the existence of hospitals was an illustration of society's failure to provide good public health for its members. One of her most famous aspirations was the hope that hospitals might one day become obsolete, adding: 'But it is no use to talk about the year 2000.'[52] Her work to reform district nursing, like her work with Poor Law hospitals, grew in part out of her friendship with the philanthropist William Rathbone. He was said to have been so impressed by the work of a nurse who cared for his wife during her final illness from consumption (tuberculosis) in 1859 that he financed a 'scheme' for district nursing in Liverpool in 1862. Known as the Liverpool Queen Victoria District Nursing Association, this was centred around a 'Nurses' Home' close to the Liverpool Royal Infirmary. Similar associations were founded in Manchester and Salford (1865), Leicester (1866), York (1870) and Glasgow (1875).[53]

The development of District Nursing Associations built upon the earlier work of religious movements such as the London Bible and Domestic Female Mission, established in 1857 and renamed the Ranyard Mission after its founder.[54] Much of the work of these early sisterhoods had been directed towards the training of nurses to care for the sick poor in their own homes, along the lines of services provided by both Protestant deaconesses and Catholic daughters of charity on the European continent. Indeed, the delivery of such care can be seen as the original raison d'etre of these organizations with the supply of nurses to hospitals as a further development of their work. In 1874, the Metropolitan and National Nursing Association for Providing Trained Nurses for the Sick Poor was launched. A nurses' home was established in Bloomsbury Square, and Florence Lees was appointed the Association's Superintendent. One of Lees's first activities was to undertake an extensive survey of existing district nursing services. Her 1874 *Report of the National Association for Providing Trained Nurses for the Sick Poor* demonstrated that a number of District Nursing Associations were operating throughout the country. Many of those based in London were employing nurses trained by institutions such as St John's House, the British Nursing Association, the East London Nursing Society and the Mildmay Park Institute.[55]

In 1887, a successful bid was made for funding from the Women's Jubilee Offering for Queen Victoria's Golden Jubilee. This enabled the foundation of the Queen Victoria Jubilee Institute for Nursing, which placed district nursing on a firm financial footing and provided an organization with which district nurses could identify. The Institute was incorporated by Royal Charter in 1889.[56] In 1890 the pioneering work of Elizabeth Malleson led to the foundation of the National Rural Nursing Association, which was affiliated to the Queen Victoria Jubilee Institute in 1891/92 and became fully amalgamated in 1897.[57] Helen Sweet claimed that by the end of the nineteenth century the roll of the Queen's Nursing Institute (QNI) contained the names of over 900 trained nurses. She also pointed out that, by this time, the required training for a Queen's District Nurse included at least one year in hospital, three months of midwifery and three to six months of training in district work.[58] Both Fox and Sweet have argued that the early twentieth century was characterized by inter-professional rivalries between district nurses and general medical practitioners, who feared that the developing new and highly professional practitioners would deprive them of patients and therefore of income.[59]

The Military Nurse

The Crimea is often seen as the birthplace of modern nursing, being inextricably linked with Nightingale's mission. However, the highly masculinized and hierarchical world of the British military was one in which female nursing found it almost impossible to gain more than a foothold;[60] and the focus of Nightingale's own post-war work was sanitary reform as it related to the health of the army and hospital design, rather than directly on the provision of a military nursing service.[61] Therefore, military nursing lagged behind civilian hospital nursing.

The Second Boer War (1899–1902) against the descendants of Dutch settlers in South Africa, which followed a brief conflict in 1881, was a pivotal influence on the development of military nursing in Britain for two reasons. Firstly, it was the first war in which a large volunteer-force was sent to swell the ranks of the regular army. This meant that when thousands of troops were killed by disease as well as by injury, their deaths aroused huge dismay throughout all classes in British society and led to outspoken demands for reform. Secondly, the need to send large numbers of civilian nurses and doctors to the conflict exposed the inadequacies of the existing military medical and nursing services.[62] Further uncertainty was created by the necessity of working closely with orderlies of the Royal Army Medical Corps, whose line of command made it, at times, difficult for nursing staff to direct their work.[63]

One of the most innovative units of the war, a field hospital formed by Frederick Treves of the London Hospital, took four trained, professional nurses to work close to the battlefields, exploding many myths of the time about the incapacity of female workers, their inability to do tough physical work or to sleep rough, and their need for servants.[64]

The efforts of campaigners and the favourable impression created by the direct hands-on work of nurses culminated in the creation of the Queen Alexandra's Imperial Military Nursing Service (QAIMNS) in 1902.[65] Its formation was governed largely by influential medical men and by Queen Alexandra herself. Nevertheless, it offered, for the first time, a clear career structure and acceptable rates of pay for army nurses. Equally innovative was the requirement that military orderlies were to work under the guidance of nursing sisters.[66]

When Britain declared war on Germany on 4 August 1914, the QAIMNS had a membership of just under 300 nurses. This was increased through the Reserve to 2,223 by the end of the year.[67] The Territorial Force Nursing Service, inaugurated in 1908, was able to augment these numbers. As had been predicted, however, there remained an acute shortage of trained nurses. Large numbers of volunteers were needed, and these were supplied by Voluntary Aid Detachments, which had been created in 1909 as part of the Territorial Force.[68] These volunteer nurses, often referred to as 'VADs', were a mixed blessing. Under the direct training and supervision of professional nurses, many became highly proficient and were able to offer valuable aid to the hard-pressed professional service. Many trained nurses, however – particularly those who were campaigning for better professional recognition through registration – were anxious that the presence of VADs within the wartime nursing services made their own thorough three-year professional training seem unnecessary and diluted standards within the profession.

Many of these fears proved unfounded. The public image of the nurse underwent an enormous boost during the war. The writings of both nurses and VADs conveyed their sense of pride in the work that they did.[69] They offered effective and often life-saving nursing care to patients suffering from serious wounds; they nursed patients with horrific infectious conditions such as gas gangrene and tetanus; they cared for the victims of attacks with toxic gases; and they offered emotional support to soldiers suffering from the notorious condition 'shell shock'.[70] Shortly after the end of the war, women and nurses made clear gains in status and recognition when in 1918 legislation that gave the parliamentary vote to women over the age of 29 was passed. Moreover, in 1919 the Nurses Registration Act was passed, creating the first professional Register for nurses.

The Professionalizing Project

The period from 1840 to 1880 has been seen as the 'pioneering age' of British nursing. After about 1880 a new era began, as the first full generation of nurses completed their training and began to look seriously for greater professional autonomy and recognition. Jane Brooks has argued for the 'divided' nature of late nineteenth- and early twentieth-century nursing. She observed that the two-tier system created by the division between 'ordinary' probationers, who were paid to both learn and work, and 'special' or 'lady' probationers, who paid a fee and could expect to be offered senior appointments on completion of their (often shortened) probationary period, meant that the profession was split along class lines between working- and middle- or upper-class members.[71]

More recently, in her 2010 publication, Sue Hawkins has argued that the hospital nursing workplace was a 'melting pot' in which women of different social classes mingled. She further demonstrated that some women used nursing as a means for social advancement, citing the example of Harriet Coster who rose from the position of a household maid to become matron of a voluntary hospital located in one of the wealthiest and most exclusive neighbourhoods of London.[72] In the 1880s, when a number of prominent middle-class members of the profession began to agitate for more robust professional status and, more particularly, for a legally recognized Register of nurses, this range of social backgrounds within the profession had an important impact on the progress of the proposed reforms.

Alongside social class – and inextricably linked with it – was the issue of the differing educational status of working-class and middle-class nurses. While many of the former had no formal education at all, the latter were often educated at home. In the mid-nineteenth century, 'ladies' were not expected to work for a living yet, towards the end of the century, as the numbers of unmarried middle-class women who needed to support themselves increased, an obvious need for paid employment (accompanied by an obvious need for formal women's education) emerged.[73] Towards the end of the nineteenth and into the twentieth century, private schools were formed for the daughters of the middle classes, which provided an education modelled, in some ways, on that received by their brothers.

Florence Nightingale had deplored the poor educational standards of some of the working-class nurses who applied to travel with her to the Crimea in 1854. Yet, at that early stage, very few educated nurses were available. In the mid-nineteenth century – before the advent of public education – it was a significant accomplishment for a working-class woman to be able to read and write. Consequently, the formation of effective training schools for nurses was a difficult and lengthy process. The Nightingale School, which is credited with being the first secular nurse training school in the world, was dogged for years by the problems of poor management and inadequate teaching. The early problems encountered by nurse-training were linked to the difficulty of knowing who should offer the teaching. Until there were educated nurses, there could be no nurse-teachers. For this reason, but also because of medical dominance within the hospitals, the lectures offered to students at St Thomas's Hospital were given by a doctor, Richard Whitfield, with guidance on their content offered by the matron and head of the Nightingale School, Sarah Wardroper. It took some time for the inadequacies of their system of training to be exposed. However, in the early 1870s, Whitfield was replaced by the surgeon, John Croft, and a former Nightingale probationer, Mary Crossland, was taken on as Home Sister, charged with the task of enabling the probationers to translate medical knowledge into nursing knowledge, and with the duty of caring for the physical, emotional and moral welfare of probationers. The role of Home Sister was a significant innovation in nurse training. It was designed both to placate the parents of middle-class girls entering nursing and to enable early probationers to begin to gain a sense of their identity as a distinct group within the hospital setting.[74]

The Nightingale School produced a number of influential nurses who took the 'Nightingale system' with them to appointments as matrons elsewhere. The enormous faith in Florence Nightingale meant that she received frequent requests to send 'teams' of nurses to reform specific hospitals. Among the most famous Nightingale 'missionaries' were Lucy Osburn, who took the British system of nursing to the Sydney Hospital in Australia; Maria Machin, who travelled as head of a group of Nightingale-nurses to Montreal, Canada; and Alice Fisher, who became matron of the Philadelphia General Hospital in the United States.[75]

It is, nevertheless, easy to over-estimate the importance of the 'Nightingale system' in the development of nursing education. Other hospitals, particularly in London, developed also their own programmes during the 1870s and 1880s. Some of these, such as the St Bartholomew's training school, under the leadership of Ethel Gordon Manson and her successor, Isla Stewart, began to develop training programmes that offered a distinctly scientific and technical training. St Bartholomew's was also the first training school to insist on three years' training for nurses.[76]

As nursing began to develop as a discipline, influential nurse leaders wrote textbooks designed to support the learning of probationers. Between the lines of these essentially practical texts, it is possible to read the ideologies being promoted by their authors. One of the earliest was co-authored by former Nightingale School probationers Rachel Williams and Alice Fisher. Their practical guide to nursing work entitled *Hints for Hospital Nurses* and published in 1877 asserted that nursing was a vocation. Their anxiety about the tendency for nursing work to become both a 'fashionable' pursuit for 'ladies' and a means of advancement for working-class women is palpable.[77]

This emphasis on nursing as a vocation or calling was very much in keeping with Florence Nightingale's perception that the essential qualities of a good nurse were moral ones, and that the nurse was primarily a 'sanitary missioner' whose role was to oversee the moral and physical well-being of her patients. These ideas were also given voice by Eva Luckes, influential matron of the London Hospital. In 1884 she published her *Lectures on General Nursing Delivered to the Probationers of the London Hospital Training School for Nurses*. This fascinating volume, which was later developed into the textbook *General Nursing*, repeatedly emphasizes the nurses' role in implementing the medical regime laid down by the doctor. But it also lays great emphasis on her moral qualities.[78]

The 'pioneers' of nursing – the leaders of the early sisterhoods, and individuals such as Florence Nightingale – developed nursing as a discipline which was based on the social mores of its own time. While the man's sphere was the world at large, the woman's was the home, and in it she exercised dominance. It was the insistence of nurse leaders in both civilian and military circles on extending this level of authority to their own staff in the hospital world that caused much of the friction between nurses and both doctors and hospital governors. Yet it was a model to which the nursing profession clung. In her *Hospital Sisters and Their Duties*, Eva Luckes commented on the superior position of the ward sister in her own domain, a superiority which she saw as almost divinely ordained.[79]

This model carried with it the assumption that the most important qualities of nursing were those that enabled excellence in domestic management and the moral guardianship of the sick. It was being challenged by the 1880s by an influential group of nurses, among whom the most prominent were Ethel Bedford Fenwick and Isla Stewart. This newly emerging generation of nurses saw the future of their profession in the development of scientific knowledge and technical skill. Isla Stewart exerted considerable influence through her textbook *Practical Nursing*, in which she made a forceful argument for the need for a strong technical education.[80]

Although co-authored with a doctor, Herbert Cuff, and emphasizing the need for the nurse to be deferential to medical authority, Stewart's textbook was one of the first to mark out a clear set of boundaries for the development of a body of knowledge that would belong to the nursing profession.

The Path to Registration

Those nurses who advocated a more scientific and technical education for their profession were also prominent among the group who in the 1880s began to campaign for a nurses' Register. Serious campaigning began with the formation of the British Nurses' Association in 1887. It was formally launched in February 1888, with Princess Christian as its President, Ethel Bedford Fenwick as its Honorary Secretary and Isla Stewart among its most influential members. It was incorporated by Royal Charter in 1893, becoming the Royal British Nurses Association (RBNA).[81] One stipulation of the new charter was that members of the Association's General Council stand for election every three years. In the succeeding elections, Ethel Bedford Fenwick and a number of other pro-registrationists lost their seats on the Council, which fell under the influence of the anti-registrationists.

In 1893, Fenwick and Stewart founded the Matron's Council, which became the main vehicle for the promotion of state registration. Among its members was the influential matron of the General Hospital, Birmingham, Ellen Musson. The Council's work led, in 1902, to the formation of the Society for the State Registration of Trained Nurses and the presentation of the first of several private members bills to parliament. In 1904 and 1905, a Parliamentary Select Committee was called to review the arguments relating to state registration. Ethel Bedford Fenwick was one of a number of vocal witnesses, arguing that the state had 'a debt of obligation to our nurses which it can only discharge by doing all in its power to organise their education and work so that they may be qualified in the best manner for the performance of their duties'.[82] The committee found in favour of state registration for nurses,[83] yet the anti-registrationists were still able to block a succession of private members bills, including one introduced by a Central Committee for the State Registration of Nurses (representing pro-registration groups from England, Scotland and Ireland) in 1910. In 1914, with the outbreak of war, the facility for private members bills was suspended, and with it the campaign for state registration.[84]

In 1916, the College of Nursing was founded in recognition that nurses needed some vehicle through which to organize themselves, develop their educational base and regulate their profession. Two distinguished individuals drove forward its creation: Sarah Swift, Matron-in-Chief of the British Red Cross (and former matron of Guy's Hospital), and Sir Arthur Stanley, politician and Chair of the British Red Cross Society. Membership was restricted to trained nurses, yet those who had founded the College were seen by Fenwick as rivals, partly because its Council included doctors and laymen as well as nurses.[85]

The essentials of the campaign for registration have been distilled to a contest between the pro-registrationists, the most prominent among whom were Ethel Bedford-Fenwick and Isla Stewart, and the anti-registrationists, represented by Eva Luckes with Florence Nightingale a shadowy background figure, never speaking publicly on the issue but clearly giving support to those who were against the formation of a Register.[86] What were the issues that drove the debates? Those in favour of a Register argued for the protection of both nurses and those they cared for against 'amateur nurses'; they insisted that permitting untrained individuals to care for patients could undermine the position of those who had been fully trained and, in a world where nursing was becoming increasingly intricate and technical, might endanger patients' lives.

The anti-registrationists had two fears. The first was that nursing would lose its moral qualities if it became a profession entered by merely passing an examination.[87] Nightingale, Luckes and those who thought like them feared that a Register would lower and not raise standards. Among Nightingale's most stinging comments was the statement that entry into a Register through the passing of examinations would turn nurses into 'mere dictionaries'.[88] The second fear driving opposition to registration arose out of the vested interest of hospital governors, particularly those who ran some of the powerful London voluntary hospitals. Influential individuals within the camp of the anti-registrationists – among whom the most prominent were probably Sydney Holland and Henry Burdett – feared a collegial nursing profession that would support the rights and demands of nurses and hence undermine the power of the hospital itself to retain its workforce and set conditions of work. In short, hospitals wished to be able to count on the undivided loyalties of 'their' nurses.[89]

Both pro- and anti-registrationists promoted their arguments through the journals over which they had editorial control. Ethel Bedford Fenwick purchased the *Nursing Record,* founded in 1888 and renamed the *British Journal of Nursing* in 1902. Henry Burdett's *Nursing Mirror* was also founded in 1888, as a section within *The Hospital.* It acted as a counter-weight to the *British Journal of Nursing*'s open and assertive campaigning for a nurses' Register.[90]

The First World War had an important impact on the fight for state registration. The experience of working with large numbers of volunteers brought home to nurses the need for some means of regulating their profession.[91] The popularity of the nursing profession was at its zenith as a result of the important work that had been done by nurses with the war-wounded. In December 1919 the Nurses Registration Act was finally passed. It has been argued that, in spite of their apparent success, following a long and sometimes bitter campaign, the pro-registrationists had little to celebrate. The Act effectively placed power in the hands of the government rather than nurses themselves, and many of its terms were drawn up by a powerful medical lobby. The ability of the profession to regulate itself was effectively limited. Pro-registrationists had hoped for a single-portal Register for the whole of Britain. What they got were three separate Registers: one for England and Wales, one for Scotland and one for Ireland; and the one Register for general nurses was accompanied by supplementary Registers for male nurses, mental health nurses, sick children's nurses and fever nurses.[92] Significantly, the formation of these supplementary Registers (along with one, slightly later, for those with a so-called 'mental deficiency') reflects an increased specialization of nursing in the twentieth century.

The creation of a 'main' Register for 'general' nurses reflects the fact that many of the political developments within the nursing profession were generated by that group. It must be noted that 'mental' nursing had followed its own powerful trajectory, with training by the Medico-Psychological Association and the creation of an Asylum Workers Union. That trajectory has not been considered in this chapter. Mental health nursing, learning disability nursing and fever nursing have complex histories of their own, which have been discussed in detail by other authors.[93]

It has been argued that the weakness of the profession – which was itself a consequence of almost incessant in-fighting – meant that nurse leaders lost the initiative in the development of their own General Council. In 1919, a Caretaker Council was put in place to draw up the new nursing Register, to decide which names might be entered into it and to compile a syllabus of training and examination for future student nurses.[94] Ethel Bedford Fenwick and her supporters were initially adamant that only nurses with training at a recognized hospital training school should be admitted to the Register. This would have meant that only a small elite could register as professional nurses. Lengthy debates led only to stalemate, and the government was forced to step in and fix the terms of entry to the Registers so that some individuals with three years' experience, but no formal training, were admitted. Commentators have observed that the divisiveness of these events and their conclusions worked against the nursing profession, undermining its strength and autonomy for decades.[95]

Conclusion

The nineteenth century can be seen as the 'era of professionalization' in nursing. It was also the era in which nursing first began to specialize. This was an extraordinary process by which the profession became much more fragmentary and divided, and through which specialisms such as physiotherapy and occupational therapy split away.

General nursing dominated these trends. Its personnel were essentially white and female. Although Mary Seacole is often 'held up' as the 'first black professional nurse', she was unique, and her example was followed by very few individuals in her own time. The social class status of general nurses has been much more debated. Some of the findings of researchers have been discussed in this chapter, which began by speculating about whether nursing can be said to have undergone a process of transformation during the nineteenth century. There can be little doubt that massive changes took place and that these altered both the structural reality and the image of the nursing profession. While claims to a seismic shift in the social class background of nurses have been largely refuted, there can be no doubt that the movement of large numbers of middle-class and more than a few upper-class individuals into the developing nursing profession had a profound influence on how it was viewed by its own members, and by society at large.

The shift in the educational status of nurses, which was, in part, a consequence of this social class shift, was probably even more profound. The burgeoning of nurse training schools during the last four decades of the century, the production of textbooks for nurses and the founding of journals dedicated to professional development provide ample evidence for the cultural shift that had taken place from a disempowered group of workers to a self-conscious profession. Once established as a 'respectable' profession for ladies, nursing began the process of carving for itself a place in the male-medical-dominated world of nineteenth- and early twentieth-century health care, both within and beyond the hospitals.

As the nineteenth century drew to a close, women's perceptions of their role in society were themselves undergoing a gradual shift as part of the emergence of the movement for woman suffrage. This gained pace in the early years of the twentieth century. Prominent campaigners for nurse registration were also often suffragists. They saw the public and political recognition of the predominantly female nursing profession as an important element of the fight for women's rights. Even for anti-suffragists almost imperceptible changes were taking place, and these found expression in the way in which nurses presented themselves to the world. Having already shifted from 'working-class Gamp' to 'self-effacing lady-nurse', nurses now shifted again to become members of a self-confident female profession.

Within a military setting, nurses fought to gain a foothold within the medical services, and yet, paradoxically, at the same time, the philanthropic efforts of wealthy and influential society ladies raised their profile. As society became increasingly 'militarized' towards the end of the nineteenth century, and as this process accelerated in the first two decades of the twentieth century, nursing became the one acceptable means by which women could play a significant role on the world stage, could act as heroines alongside their soldier-brothers and could demonstrate their right to citizenship-status. The self-denying 'lady nurse' of the Crimea had given way to the heroic professional military nurse of the early twentieth century. In 1919 the drives for reform and autonomy came together as the creation of a State Register for nurses recognized the need for professional self-regulation, for uniform standards of care and for an adequate and effectively tested system of education. Nursing had travelled a long way from the days of 'Sarah Gamp' and 'Betsy Prig'. By creating a Register, gaining public esteem and respect, and developing a disciplinary body of knowledge, its members had succeeded in forging themselves into a recognized and respected profession.

Acknowledgement

The author would like to acknowledge the financial support of the Nursing and Midwifery Council, UK, for some of the research work for this chapter.

Notes

1. S. Tooley, *The History of Nursing in the British Empire* (London, S.H. Bousefield and Co, 1906); L.R. Seymer, *A General History of Nursing* (London, Faber and Faber Ltd, 1949); M.A. Nutting and L.L. Dock, *A History of Nursing*, vols I and II (New York and London, G.P. Putnam's Sons, 1907); L. Dock, *The History of Nursing*, vols III and IV (New York and London, G.P. Putnam's Sons, 1912); M. Goodnow, *Outlines of Nursing History* (Philadelphia, W.B. Saunders, 1923).

2. B. Mortimer, 'Independent Women: Domiciliary Nurses in Mid-Nineteenth-Century Edinburgh', in A.M. Rafferty, J. Robinson and R. Elkan (eds), *Nursing History and the Politics of Welfare* (London: Routledge, 1997) pp. 133–49.

3. A. Summers, 'The Mysterious Demise of Sarah Gamp: The Domiciliary Nurse and Her Detractors c.1830–1860', *Victorian Studies*, 32:3 (1989) 365–86.

4. A.M. Rafferty, *The Politics of Nursing Knowledge* (London: Routledge, 1996) p. 13.

5. L. McDonald, *Florence Nightingale at First Hand* (London: Continuum, 2010) p. 107; C. Helmstadter, ' "A Real Tone": Professionalizing Nursing in Nineteenth-Century London', *Nursing History Review*, 11 (2003) 3–30.

6. R. White, *Social Change and the Development of the Nursing Profession: A Study of the Poor Law Nursing Service 1848–1948* (London: Henry Kimpton Publishers, 1978) pp. 20–2, 30; S. Hawkins, *Nursing and Women's Labour in the Nineteenth Century: The Quest for Independence* (London: Routledge, 2010) pp. 18–20.

7. A. Simnett, 'The Pursuit of Respectability: Women and the Nursing Profession, 1860–1900', in R. White (ed.), *Political Issues in Nursing: Past Present and Future*, vol. 2 (Chichester: John Wiley and Sons, 1986) p. 9.

8. P. Nolan, *A History of Mental Health Nursing* (Cheltenham: Stanley Thornes, 1998).

9. A. Summers, *Angels and Citizens: British Women as Military Nurses 1854–1914*, revised edn (London: Routledge and Kegan Paul, 1988).

10. E. Gamarnikow, 'Nurse or Woman: Gender and Professionalism in Reformed Nursing, 1860–1923', in P. Holden and J. Littlewood (eds), *Anthropology and Nursing* (London: Routledge, 1991) pp. 110–29. See also: E. Gamarnikow, 'Women's Employment and the Sexual Division of Labour: The Case of Nursing', in A. Kuhn and A. Wolpe (eds), *Feminism and Materialism: Women and Modes of Production* (London: Routledge and Kegan Paul, 1978) pp. 98–123; A. Bashford, *Purity and Pollution: Gender, Embodiment and Victorian Medicine* (Basingstoke: Macmillan, 1998); L. Davidoff, 'Class and Gender in Victorian England', in J. Newton, M. Ryan and J. Walkowitz (eds), *Sex and Class in Women's History* (London: Routledge and Kegan Paul, 1983) pp. 16–71.

11. M. Vicinus, *Independent Women: Work and Community for Single Women, 1850–1920* (London: Virago Press, 1985).

12. S. Nelson, *Say Little, Do Much: Nursing, Nuns and Hospitals in the Nineteenth Century* (Philadelphia: University of Pennsylvania Press, 2001) p. 56.

13. Nelson, *Say Little*, pp. 60–5. On Catholic communities, see also: C. Mangion, *Contested Identities: Catholic Women Religious in Nineteenth Century England and Wales* (Manchester: Manchester University Press, 2008).

14. R.G. Huntsman, M. Bruin and D. Holttum, 'Twixt Candle and Lamp: The Contribution of Elizabeth Fry and the Institution of Nursing Sisters to Nursing Reform', *Medical History*, 46:3 (2002) 351–80.

15. Nelson, *Say Little*, p. 66

16. Vicinus, *Independent Women*; Nelson, *Say Little*, pp. 67–70.

17. A. Summers, 'The Cost and Benefits of Caring: Nursing Charities, c.1830–1860', in J. Barry and C. Jones (eds), *Medicine and Charity before the Welfare State* (London: Routledge, 1991) pp. 133–48; Nelson, *Say Little*, pp. 70–1.

18. J.A.G. Widerquist, 'Dearest Friend. The Correspondence of Colleagues Florence Nightingale and Mary Jones', *Nursing History Review*, 1 (1993) 25–42.

19. J. Moore, *A Zeal for Responsibility: The Struggle for Professional Nursing in Victorian England, 1868–1883* (Athens: The University of Georgia Press, 1988). See also: C. Helmstadter, 'Robert Bentley Todd, St John's

House and the Origins of the Modern Trained Nurse', *Bulletin of the History of Medicine*, 67 (1993) 282–319; C. Helmstadter, 'Nurse Recruitment and Retention in the 19th Century London Teaching Hospitals', *International History of Nursing Journal* 2:1 (1992) 58–69, 62–4.

20. Nelson, *Say Little,* pp. 71–5.
21. Nelson, *Say Little,* p. 74.
22. The best-known biographies of Nightingale are E. Cooke, *The Life of Florence Nightingale* (London: Macmillan, 1913); S. Tooley, *The Life of Florence Nightingale* (London: S.H. Bousefield, 1904); L. Strachey, *Eminent Victorians* (Oxford: Oxford University Press, 1918); B. Dossey, *Florence Nightingale: Mystic, Visionary, Healer* (Pennsylvania: Springhouse, 2000); Bostridge, *Florence Nightingale: The Woman and Her Legend* (London: Viking/Penguin, 2008).
23. F. Nightingale, *Notes on Nursing: What It Is and What It Is Not* (Edinburgh, Churchill Livingstone, 1980 edition) p. 2.
24. M. Bostridge, Florence Nightingale, pp. 54–5, 142–6, 183–4, 202–11; C. Helmstadter, 'Navigating the Political Straits in the Crimean War', in S. Nelson and A.M. Rafferty (eds), Notes on Nightingale: The Influence and Legacy of a Nursing Icon (Ithaca: Cornell University Press, 2010) pp. 28–54.
25. M. Baly, *Florence Nightingale and the Nursing Legacy*, 2nd edn (London: Whurr, 1997) pp. 20–66. On the Nightingale School, see L. McDonald (ed.), *Florence Nightingale: The Nightingale School*, vol. 12, Collected Works of Florence Nightingale (Waterloo, Ontario, Canada: Wilfrid Laurier University Press, 2009).
26. L. McDonald, 'Mythologizing and De-mythologizing', in S. Nelson and A.M. Rafferty (eds), *Notes on Nightingale*, pp. 91–114; L. McDonald (ed.), *Florence Nightingale: Extending Nursing*, vol. 13, Collected Works of Florence Nightingale (Waterloo, Ontario, Canada: Wilfrid Laurier University Press, 2009).
27. Baly, *Florence Nightingale*, p. 124.
28. E. Parker and S. Collins, *Learning to Care: A History of Nursing and Midwifery Education at the Royal London Hospital, 1740–1993* (London: Royal London Hospital Archives and Museum, 1998) p. 18.
29. C. Davies (ed.), *Rewriting Nursing History* (London: Croom Helm, 1980) frontispiece, p. 11; Rafferty, *Politics*.
30. C. Maggs, *The Origins of General Nursing* (London: Croom Helm, 1983); Hawkins, *Nursing*.
31. Helmstadter, 'Nurse Recruitment and Retention', pp. 61–2.
32. C. Helmstadter, ' "A Real Tone": Professionalizing Nursing in Nineteenth-Century London', *Nursing History Review*, 11 (2003) 5, 7–8.
33. Helmstadter, 'A Real Tone', p. 24.
34. Simnett, 'Pursuit', pp. 3–8.

35. L. Lynn McDonald (ed.) *Florence Nightingale: The Nightingale School*, vol. 12, Collected Works of Florence Nightingale (Waterloo, Ontario, Canada: Wilfrid Laurier University Press, 2009) pp. 8–10.
36. Moore, *Zeal*, passim.
37. Moore, *Zeal*, p. 55.
38. M. Lonsdale, 'The Present Crisis at Guy's Hospital', *The Nineteenth Century* (7 April 1880) 677–78; Moore, *Zeal*, pp. 55, 74–97; A. Pringle and J. Bell, *Nurses and Doctors: Reprinted (by permission) from the 'Edinburgh Medical Journal', May, 1880, for the Council of the Nightingale Fund* (London: Nightingale Fund, 1880); A. Pringle, *A Study in Nursing* (London: Macmillan, 1905).
39. Moore, *Zeal*, pp. 55–74.
40. Moore, *Zeal*, pp. 75–97; M. Baly, 'The Lonsdale Affair: A Nineteenth Century Struggle for Nurse Power', *History of Nursing Society Journal*, 4 (4) (1992/3); A. Knight, 'The Great Nursing Dispute of Guy's Hospital 1979–1880', *International History of Nursing Journal*, 3:1 (1997), 52–68; K. Waddington, 'The Nursing Dispute at Guy's 1879–1880', *Social History of Medicine* 8 (1995) pp. 211–30.
41. A. Pringle and J. Bell, *Nurses and Doctors: Reprinted (by permission) from the 'Edinburgh Medical Journal' May, 1880, for the Council of the Nightingale Fund* (London: Nightingale Fund, 1880), available at the London Metropolitan Archives H01/ST/NC16/10; A. Pringle, *A Study in Nursing* (London: Macmillan and Co. Ltd, 1905), available at the London Metropolitan Archives H01/ST/NC/16/6; O. Sturges, S.J. Starkey; M. Lonsdale 'Doctors and Nurses', *The Nineteenth Century*, vol. VII (June 1880) pp. 1089–108.
42. Nurse Ingle was convicted of manslaughter and imprisoned. See London Metropolitan Archives; Guy's Hospital; papers and correspondence relating to patient alleged to be ill treated in 'Mary' Ward, July 1880; H09/GY/A231/1 and 2; Guy's Hospital; papers relating to the public prosecution of Louisa Ingle, August 1880; H09/GY/A231/8; and A232/1; and A230/3.
43. C. Maggs, *The Origins of General Nursing* (London: Croom Helm, 1983) pp. 2, 21, 146–147.
44. White, *Social Change*.
45. Baly, *Florence Nightingale*, p. 87.
46. Bostridge, *Florence Nightingale*, pp. 426–7.
47. Bostridge, *Florence Nightingale*, pp. 420–3
48. L. McDonald (ed.), *Florence Nightingale on Public Health Care*, vol. 6, Collected Works of Florence Nightingale (Waterloo, Ontario, Canada: Wilfrid Laurier University Press, 2004) p. 249.
49. McDonald (ed.), *Florence Nightingale: Extending Nursing*, pp. 93–100.
50. McDonald (ed.), *Florence Nightingale on Public Health Care*, pp. 278–80.

51. White, *Social Change;* G. Rivett, *The Development of the London Hospital System, 1823–1982* (London: The King's Fund, 1986); A.C. Gibson, *Nursing in Workhouses and Workhouse Infirmaries. A Paper Read at the Central Poor Law Conference Held at the Guildhall, London, February 13th, 1895 by A.C. Gibson, Matron of the Birmingham Workhouse Infirmary* (London: Knight and Co, 1895).

52. Baly, *Florence Nightingale*, p. 121, citing a letter from Nightingale to Henry Bonham Carter dated 4 June 1867.

53. H. Sweet with R. Dougall, *Community Nursing and Primary Healthcare in Twentieth-Century Britain* (London: Routledge, 2008) p. 20.

54. L. Williamson, 'Soul Sisters: The St John and Ranyard nurses in Nineteenth-Century London', *International History of Nursing Journal*, 2:2 (1996) 33–49; F.K. Prochaska, 'Body and Soul: Bible Nurses and the Poor in Victorian London', *Historical Research*, 60:143 (1987) 336–48; M. Stocks, *A Hundred Years of District Nursing* (London: Allen and Unwin, 1960) p. 25.

55. Baly, *Florence Nightingale*, pp. 124–6; Sweet with Dougall, *Community Nursing*, pp. 18, 21–5; M. Baly, *A History of the Queen's Nursing Institute: 100 Years 1887–1987* (London: Croom Helm, 1987) pp. 12–16.

56. Sweet with Dougall, *Community Nursing*, p. 21; Baly, *Florence Nightingale*, p. 130; Baly, *History*, pp. 18–32.

57. C. Howse, *Rural District Nursing in Gloucestershire, 1880–1925* (Cheltenham: Reardon, 2008) p. 8; Baly, *History*, pp. 48–60.

58. Sweet with Dougall, *Community Nursing*, p. 25.

59. E. Fox, 'District Nursing Associations and Doctors: Aspects of Inter-Professional Relationships, 1902–1914', *International History of Nursing Journal*, 1:3 (1996) 18–33; Sweet, with Dougall, *Community Nursing*, pp. 26–30.

60. Summers, *Angels*, pp. 67–96.

61. Bostridge, *Florence Nightingale*, pp. 312, 316–17, 336; Helmstadter, 'Navigating', pp. 28–54; J. Piggott, *Queen Alexandra's Royal Army Nursing Corps* (London: Leo Cooper Ltd, 1975) pp. 18–19.

62. Summers, *Angels*, pp. 29–66; Bostridge, *Florence Nightingale*, pp. 215–300.

63. See, for example, E. Laurence, *A Nurse's Life in War and Peace,* (London, 1912); Guy's Hospital Gazette obituary of Eleanor Constance Lawrence [*sic*]; 18 January 1912; Available at London Metropolitan Archives; H09/GY/C/05/001/004.

64. Summers, *Angels*, pp. 211–18.

65. Piggott, *Queen Alexandra's Royal Army Nursing Corps*, pp. 37–40.

66. Summers, *Angels*, pp. 220–31.

67. Piggott, *Queen Alexandra's Royal Army Nursing Corps*; I. Hay, *One Hundred Years of Army Nursing* (London: Cassel and Company, 1953); E. Taylor, *Wartime Nurse: One Hundred Years from the Crimea to Korea, 1854–1954* (London: Robert Hale, 2001).

68. Summers, *Angels*, pp. 238–70.
69. Particularly vivid descriptions of nursing work are offered by trained professional nurses. See, for example, K. Luard, *Unknown Warriors: Extracts from the Letters of K. E. Luard, RRC, Nursing Sister in France, 1914–1918* (London: Chatto and Windus, 1930); V. Thurstan, *Field Hospital and Flying Column: Being the Journal of an English Nursing Sister in Belgium and Russia* (London: G.P. Putnam's Sons, 1915). Large numbers of unpublished diaries also exist in archives such as the Imperial War Museum, London. See, for example, M.A. Brown, 'Diaries, May 1915–January 1918', 1001, 88/7/1; Mary Clarke, 'MS Diary'; 84/46/1; Lily Doughty-Wylie, 'Twenty-six MS diaries', 6665, 79/37/2.
70. Christine Hallett, *Containing Trauma: Nursing Work in the First World War* (Manchester: Manchester University Press, 2009).
71. J. Brooks, 'Structured by Class, Bound by Gender: Nursing and Special Probationer Schemes, 1860–1939', *International History of Nursing Journal*, 6:2 (2001) 13–21.
72. Hawkins, *Nursing*, p. 34.
73. Hawkins, *Nursing*, p. 34.
74. Papers of the Nightingale School; London Metropolitan Archives A/NFC; H01/ST/NC; McDonald (ed.), *Florence Nightingale: The Nightingale School*, pp. 8–11.
75. McDonald (ed.), *Florence Nightingale: Extending Nursing*.
76. I. Stewart and H. Cuff, *Practical Nursing*, 4 vols (Edinburgh: William Blackwood and Sons, 1899–1903). See also S. McGann, *The Battle of the Nurses: A Study of Eight Women Who Influenced the Development of Professional Nursing, 1880–1930* (London: Scutari Press, 1992).
77. R. Norris, *Hints for Hospital Nurses, Arranged by R. Williams and A. Fisher* (www.General-Books.net, General Books, 2009, reproduction of book published in 1877).
78. E. Luckes, *Lectures on General Nursing Delivered to the Probationers of the London Hospital Training School for Nurses* (London: Kegan Paul, Trench and Co, 1884). See also: E. Luckes, *General Nursing*. New and Revised (Ninth) Edition (London: Kegan Paul, Trench, Trubner and Co, Ltd, 1914).
79. E. Luckes, *Hospital Sisters and Their Duties*, American edn (Philadelphia: P. Blakiston, Son and Co, 1886) pp. 2–3.
80. Stewart and Cuff, *Practical Nursing*, vol. 1, pp. 4–5.
81. McGann, *Battle*, pp. 38–9; Summers, *Angels*, p. 182.
82. *Report from the Select Committee on Registration of Nurses* (London: HMSO, 1905), minutes of evidence taken from Mrs Ethel Gordon Fenwick, p. 32.
83. Officially, there were two select committees, each of which produced a separate report: *Report from the Select Committee on Registration of Nurses* (London: HMSO, 1904); *Report from the Select Committee on Registration*

of *Nurses* (London: HMSO, 1905). See also B. Abel-Smith, *A History of the Nursing Profession,* (London: Heinemann, 1960) p. 79.

84. McGann, *Battle,* pp. 4–5; E. Bendall and E. Raybould, *A History of the General Nursing Council for England and Wales, 1919–1969* (London: H.K. Lewis and Co. Ltd, 1969) pp. 1–26.

85. S. McGann, A. Crowther and R. Dougall, *A Voice for Nurses: A History of the Royal College of Nursing, 1916–1990* (Manchester: Manchester University Press, 2009) pp. 5, 9.

86. Abel-Smith, *History*; McGann, *Battle*; Bendall and Raybould, *History*; Rafferty, *Politics*.

87. McGann, *Battle,* p. 25.

88. Bostridge, *Florence Nightingale.* Some of Nightingale's supporters and associates were quite vocal opponents of nurse registration: H. Bonham-Carter, *Is a General Register for Nurses Desirable* (London: Blades, East and Blades, 1888); available at London Metropolitan Archives H01/ST/NC/16/11; H. Bonham-Carter, *Suggestions for Improving the Management of Nursing Departments in Large Hospitals* (London: Blades, East and Blades, 1867); London Metropolitan Archives; H01/ST/NC/16.

89. McGann, *Battle,* p. 3.

90. McGann, *Battle,* p. 39. A third significant nursing journal, the *Nursing Times,* was founded in 1905.

91. Abel-Smith, *History,* pp. 83–7.

92. *A Bill to Provide for the State Registration of Nurses, AD 1919* (London: HMSO, 1919); available at the National Archives, Kew, 'Registrar's Reference Papers', DT2/2. For commentary, see McGann, *Battle,* p. 6.

93. P. Nolan, *A History of Mental Health Nursing* (London: Nelson Thornes, 2000); M. Currie, *Fever Hospitals and Fever Nurses* (London: Routledge, 2005); D. Mitchell and A.M. Rafferty, ' "I don't think they ever really wanted to know anything about us": Staff Stories in Institutions for People with Learning Disability', *Oral History* (Spring 2005), 77–87.

94. The National Archives, DT2/1, 'Draft Rules' drawn up for nurses under the GNC. For an overview, see Bendall and Raybould, *History,* pp. 38–67.

95. 'Registrar's Reference Files'; available at The National Archives Dt2/3 Parts 1 and 2; also DT2/4. The dispute over the registration of 'untrained' nurses can be viewed at: 'Rule 9 (1) (g) Dr Chapple's Amendment'; The National Archives DT 2/5; Abel-Smith, *History,* pp. 83–7; McGann, *Battle.*

4

Nursing, 1920–2000: The Dilemmas of Professionalization

Andrew Hull with Andrea Jones

This chapter will focus on the dilemmas created by ongoing attempts to professionalize nursing, their contexts and consequences. The key themes will be competing concepts of professionalization, educational and managerial; the new structures and cultures of health-care systems, especially the link between nurse education and the needs of management and service; and the perils of de-professionalization. The development of the professional nurse will be examined in three key periods: between 1920–49, when the post-Registration Act schism over who was a 'nurse' gave way to wartime unity, facilitating the move into a corporatist National Health Service (NHS) structure and culture; between 1950–86, when new nurse leaders emerged and developed distinctive professional models; and between 1986–2000, when nurses constructed fully fledged but fatally flawed professionalization strategies as academics and managers.

Nurses, along with social workers, teachers and other health-care workers, can usefully be understood as 'insecure professionals'. Whereas prestigious professions (such as medicine) were helped by the state to establish and maintain their jurisdictions while preserving autonomy, insecure professions struggled to establish discrete areas of expertise and social usefulness, and were often subjected to politically motivated state control. In examining such proto-professions, rather than look for the traditional sociological markers of professional status, we need, as Nottingham suggests, to 'focus on the political struggle for jurisdiction'.[1] From 1920 to 2000, the questions of what 'professional' nursing should be, and what 'adequate' training was, were endlessly debated in attempts to stake out a meaningful claim to a specialized health-care expertise. Nursing pursued this elusive professional status, based on the model of medical professionalization. In the changing institutional and administrative structures and cultures of the expanding state health-care system, the traditional unified influence of the matron was broken down into discrete areas. Nurses had to find new ways to articulate a distinctive professional expertise and identity. Different professionalizing groups emerged, which planned to produce new elite cadres of nurses. These elite nurses would, by virtue of their specialized expertise, achieve professional autonomy from medicine and other health-care workers and define and control nursing, and perhaps wider health policy.[2] However, these competing professionalizing strategies re-ignited long-standing internal ideological differences about the nature and scope of nursing dating back to Florence Nightingale and Ethel Bedford Fenwick. Was nursing vocational, a matter of innate moral character and practical art, or a teachable technical or managerial science? Were good nurses born or made?

In framing these competing strategies, nurse leaders hoped to free nursing from the constraining identity imposed by the dominant social forces that constructed it: medicine, the state and gender. Doctors feared encroachment on their professional domain, and the state – which increasingly used medical expertise to implement health and welfare policies – backed them. In any case, there had to be nurses for the increasingly state-run hospitals to function and so strict control of nursing roles and numbers was embedded in the system. So too was a pernicious sexism that has consistently viewed nursing work as (no more than) women's work. Necessarily unskilled and essentially untheorizable, it was simply the extension to a limited public sphere of the natural female nurturing instincts.[3]

The linkage between nursing's professional development and medicine meant nursing became increasingly dominated by hospital-based models. There was a shift in the main locus of care from community to hospital, with rising hospital usage; but more than that general nursing in hospitals became the professional template.[4] Nursing care became increasingly important to twentieth-century hospital practice, especially to patients' experiences. As advancing medicine grew more impersonal and corporatist in the emerging welfare state's mass health-care system – its knowledge and practice reductionist, and its systems bureaucratized[5] – nursing expanded to fill the human-shaped gap in care. As the most influential UK nursing textbook argued in 1938, echoing the vocationalist ethos of selfless service:

> The latest advances in Medical Science are brought to the bedside by the doctor, let the nurse see that her part is to provide, in full measure, the healing touch of human sympathy. The smallest service done to the lowliest possesses an eternal value.[6]

Reflecting the pursuit of professional autonomy, by 1967 the text argued for a stronger scientific role for nursing: 'the nurse collaborating'[7] in bringing bench to bedside. In 1980 Virginia Henderson wrote in a new foreword that, while the function of nursing was to create the conditions for healing, there was now also a key 'role for the nurse that demands independence of thought and action' in its determination and delivery.[8]

However, shadowing medicine's professional trajectory was divisive. The unifying ethos of holistic nursing itself defined nursing as starting where medicine chose to end. Moreover, many rank-and-file nurses felt that their leaders had betrayed those core humanistic values of nursing in a Faustian professional bargain, as basic nursing was increasingly relegated to subsidiary grades. At the same time, many nursing groups felt alienated from unified, hospital-based conceptions of nurses as highly educated and specialized technical practitioners/managers, while nurse educators increasingly felt that academic nursing curricula were increasingly distanced from practice.[9]

1920–49: A Unified and Unitary Profession?

After the 1919 Registration Act, nurses still remained divided; chiefly by where they worked, though this also often embodied other divisions. Voluntary hospital nurses (especially from teaching hospitals) tended to be of a higher social status, whereas Poor Law hospital nurses (and municipal nurses after 1929) were of a lower social and educational standing. In the community, district nurses were usually working-class women,[10] while in asylums, nurses were mostly lower-class men. Moreover, men were not allowed onto the general Register. Male, mental deficiency, children's and other specialist nurses (e.g. fever, tuberculosis) had separate supplementary Registers. However, nurse leaders in voluntary hospitals, the matron-dominated

College of Nursing (which gained its Royal Charter in 1928) and the General Nursing Council (GNC) behaved as if all nurses were, or should be, educated, middle-class women. This necessarily alienated other nursing groups, driving them into the willing arms of the emerging nursing trade unions, whose focus on pay and conditions further reinforced their distance from emerging professional identities. Furthermore, nurse leaders themselves continued to be divided between the supporters of general training and a practical, vocational ethos, and those supporting specialist education and a professional ethos.[11]

These divisions led to the extreme inertia of the early years of the GNC, and the problems of premature professionalization, as the professionalizers attempted to limit access by setting the criteria for entry to education and the nursing Register higher than the current female take-up of secondary education would allow.[12] The resulting nurse shortages exposed the limited nature of self-regulation, as the state stepped in to ensure the provision of the numbers needed by the medical services.

In the 1920s, the GNC had power to define what constituted core nursing skills and attributes, but was divided and uncertain about the nature and scope of its role. The period of the Registration Act may have been the only point in the twentieth century when there were enough nurses; but the Voluntary Aid Detachments or VAD nurses went home, and suddenly there was an acute nursing shortage that became a chronic condition. Although absolute supply continuously increased, except during economic depressions, demand for nurses (both trained and untrained) kept outstripping it, partly because of changes in medicine (e.g. as increasing use of technology meant more intricate procedures and larger operative teams) and in the delivery of medical services.

In the interwar period, the majority of nurses were un- or undertrained and stayed unregistered. By 1925, only 28,000 of the 120,000 nurses on the Register had met the searching requirements of the GNC, although around a third had probably completed a year's approved hospital training.[13] Given increasing demand, hospitals (plus private and community work) relied on nurses with no, or less than three years, training. Moreover, even in 1937, only 28,000 girls per year were educated to target secondary level. The Athlone Committee estimated in 1939 that nursing must attract about 12,000 of these to maintain staffing levels, and it was increasingly competing with other female occupations. Nurse leaders had to navigate between the

Scylla and Charybdis of nursing shortage and state regulation, and educational dilution and the loss of the war-won proto-professional status. For years the major fear was that splitting into subsidiary grades would fatally weaken the claim to professional status, based as it was, like medicine's, on unity in diversity.[14]

Riven by faction over conditions for Register entry, the GNC set them unrealistically high (1 year of training, or 19 of service). Parliament intervened, passing Dr Chapple's amendment in July 1923, which allowed a general nurse with three years of clinical experience (attested by two doctors) and competent nursing knowledge (attested by a registered nurse *and* two doctors) to be accepted for registration; the rule did not apply to men. Here was a firm assertion of patriarchy in both its governmental and medical forms. Nurses continued in-fighting over a mandatory curriculum – a moderate one with scientific, social and practical subjects aimed at developing 'an efficient machine at the expense of the vitalizing spirit [to] develop the *mind* as well as the *heart* and *hand*'[15] – but this was blocked by the Minister of Health. Since nurse education was inextricably bound to service needs, the interwar state had increasingly strong interests in ensuring an adequate supply of nurses, and strong disincentives to disturbing the *status quo*. Nursing was expected to adjust to healthcare service reforms without any synchronized or systematic review of the impacts on nursing. As Rafferty has argued, it was most often the state that shaped nursing educational policy, not nurses.[16]

However, the new educationalists continued to pursue their agenda. In 1918, the College of Nursing had launched its Sister Tutor Certificate course at King's College for Women.[17] Increased links between College Council and London University led to an extra-mural Nursing Diploma from 1925. Covering basic medical sciences, preventive and social medicine, social psychology and modern nursing developments, it became the main qualification for ambitious nurses wishing to enter embryonic educational and managerial elites.[18] The 1928 Royal Charter committed the College to education as a core activity, and in 1930 an Educational Department was established. Training a cadre of Sister Tutors became the preserve of the Royal College of Nursing (RCN) until the 1950s, creating an emergent group of nurse educationalists who developed national educational ambitions and strategies, and also raising probationer/registration educational standards. However, training content and length remained controversial, reopening rifts in the nascent profession in the 1930s between supporters of practical clinical training and the pro-academicization lobby.[19]

The latter wanted secondary school education for all those entering nurse training. Although matrons complained of falling educational standards, nursing was taking a larger proportion of better-educated women;[20] but could this upward trend be maintained sufficiently to create an entirely educationally elite profession? Although there was no drop in the number of recruits, both the *Lancet* (1932) and Athlone (1937) Committees found evidence of nursing shortage, due to an exponential increase in demand. Given the low relative take-up of female secondary education, educationalist recruitment aims were unrealistic – like their earlier overambitious attempts to set entry criteria, and the nursing syllabus; too much was being attempted too quickly. The shortage meant that hospitals, especially small and chronic sickness ones, simply employed more unregistered nursing staff, undermining the idea of a unified elite profession in which all who did nursing work were registered nurses. Municipal hospitals used nursing orderlies for domestic work, and Essex County Council pioneered an assistant nurse training scheme, soon copied by other local authorities. RCN adhered fixedly to the one-portal principle, fearing dilution and threats to professional status, but the British Medical Association and the Athlone Committee warned that, since a subordinate grade would always be necessary, it was better under professional jurisdiction. Athlone also scotched the myth of middle-class recruitment: as in the late nineteenth century, most nurses came from the lower middle and respectable working classes – women who might also become clerks, typists and shop assistants.[21]

It was Poor Law, municipal and other local authority hospital nurses, perhaps threatened by some county councils' increasing use of subsidiary grades, who mostly joined the new nursing unions (such as the Guild of Nurses and the Professional Union of Trained Nurses) which were increasingly active in the 1930s. There was a series of negotiations between the hospital management committees of the municipal hospitals, the unions and RCN about the introduction of a 48-hour working week, in which the College was labelled 'an organization of voluntary snobs' by student nurses, reflecting widespread perceptions that it was out of touch with the grass roots. The unionization issue again challenged the College's idea of a unified professionalization strategy. Were general nurses more like other types of nurses than they were like general workers? Should nursing aim at being a unified profession or should each branch form its own professional organizations (as mental health nurses had done)?[22]

The Second World War fuelled the development of corporate state health care, notably through the national Emergency Medical Services (EMS). In nursing, similarly, the war catalyzed the central organization of nursing services, and the second portal for subordinate grade nurses. The Civil Nursing Reserve employed Assistant Nurses; from 1941, new entrants had to have two years of hospital training (not necessarily in GNC-approved institutions). In 1943, the Rushcliffe Committee published a separate salary scale for assistants, and hospital management committees increasingly pressed for professional recognition and a clear definition of the new grade. When RCN established the Horder Reconstruction Committee in 1941, first on the agenda were assistant nurses, now presented as integral – a guarantor of the advanced professional status of the State registered nurse (SRN). A separate 'Roll' for assistant nurses formed part of the 1943 Nurses Act.[23]

However, nurse shortages continued, in spite of the Minister of Health's suspension of minimum educational requirements in 1938: a suspension that lasted until 1962. In other ways, the Ministry actually supported the educationalist's professionalization strategy. The Athlone Report had recommended that student status mean a proper balance between ward work and theoretical study time, and the second Horder Report (1943) urged rationalization and inspection of small schools. The Ministry's 1946 (Wood) Nurse Recruitment and Training Working Party went much further. Mindful of NHS nursing organization and staffing levels, Wood was a concerted attack on matron-control: an apologia for modern, academic education. The Report wanted to remove the GNC's educational role, reducing it to an examining body, arguing that, unlike the GMC, it had little educational/academic representation. Wood recommended Regional Nurse Training Councils to run new, independent training schools, but the matron-dominated GNC and RCN responses were hostile and failed to understand (or rejected) the professional autonomy on offer. While the educationally progressive 'Ten Group'[24] of nurses, influenced by US educational methods, wanted broad-ranging degree preparation for expanded NHS roles and a nursing research seedbed, the traditional matron elite successfully defended the old system. As White argued: 'Once again the service interests of the profession overruled the interests of education ... the matrons' interests ... were directly antithetical to the development of the profession.'[25] Nothing more clearly underscores the interdependence between voluntary hospital matrons, doctors and the state, and their mutual interest in preserving the *status quo*, than this rejection of educational independence. The *Nursing Times* warned that loss of matron-control 'will produce the type of nurse teacher who is interested in nurse education, but is not interested in the hospitals and the nursing service that they provide'.[26] As Miss MacManus, Guy's Hospital matron, argued, nursing was more practical art than science; 'whilst the profession did not want the dunce with clever hands, American methods led her to consider nursing more an exploration into medicine'.[27]

This intense opposition influenced the 1949 Nurses Act; education was left untouched in a general housekeeping exercise synchronizing nurse education's financial and administrative organization with NHS structures, underlining central Ministry control. No fundamental consideration had been given to nursing's place within the NHS, yet the traditional hospital-orientated systems were wholly unfitted for the new regionality.[28]

1950–86: Professionalization, Nursing Hierarchies and Nurse Education

Further developments were facilitated, however, by the changing nature of the nursing elite. Many of those appointed to the newly elected GNC in 1950 represented a new generation in nursing leadership, socialized into the priorities and culture of the new health service. Many had entered the profession after the lifting of the minimum entry requirement; to them NHS service needs were increasingly more important than creating a higher class, more educated profession.[29] When, in 1962, the minimum entry requirement was re-introduced at the low level of two O levels, the GNC effectively became the implementer of state health manpower policy, relinquishing its educational role.[30] However, the RCN took it up with re-doubled commitment. The scene was set for the transformation of the old vocational/organizational versus professional/educational debate into a new form. In the new NHS structures and culture, in which business general management was increasingly prized as the tool of rational decision-making, and in which medical education was synchronized around a central university teaching hospital, nurse leaders began to develop distinct professionalization strategies that emphasized nursing as defined by specialized educational or managerial expertise.

This bifurcation of professionalization strategies was exacerbated by the increasing reduction in, and fragmentation of, the matron's role in the new NHS structures and culture. The matron had been head of a hospital's nurse training school, responsible for the nursing service on the wards and also an executive administrative officer, and was often called upon to make decisions outside of her own professional area. She had combined supreme authority over the majority of female hospital staff (e.g. nurses, cleaners, physical and radio-therapists), although remaining subservient to medical authority. Moreover, she had integrated authority over the total patient experience. However, this unified educational and managerial role was dis-integrated, especially after 1948, by bureaucratizing and specializing tendencies within the new health-care system. Matrons were not included (and were rarely represented) on the new Hospital Management Committees or Regional Hospital Boards, lost oversight of all extra-nursing staff, and even some direct control over nurse training. As the GNC closed smaller schools and created aggregated group schools, many matrons lost school headships and thus the teaching of their own students. By the 1950s, the now more prevalent Senior Nurse Tutors, influenced by American models, were becoming educationalists, taking increasing control of a curriculum that included sociology and psychology, and thus edging out the matrons in the new educational hierarchy. Matrons' sphere of influence was reduced from general hospital policy to the nursing service, narrowly defined. As a consequence, the status of nursing itself declined, as that of administrators rose. At HMC and RHB level, administrators increasingly protected their growing authority by excluding nurses, even when instructed to include them by the Ministry.[31]

As the matron's role was dis-integrated, the individual fragments took on professional lives of their own; new competing identities and strategies for the professional development of nursing began to coalesce around new versions of traditional internal divisions about the nature and scope of nursing. Thus the two competing ideologies of the 'moral-vocational' versus the 'educational-professional' now became the educated, specialist nurse, and the nurse as manager.

In the 1950s, more young women were staying on at school and choosing nursing. The 1951 census recorded 225,000 nurses, of which 130,000 (60 per cent) worked in hospitals, yet the nurse shortage continued, partly due to staffing-level increases and reductions in working hours.[32] Shortages again led to recruitment of un/under-qualified nurses. By 1958, unqualified staff outnumbered State Enrolled (i.e. assistant) Nurses (SENs) by 2:1, making up 25 per cent

of the nursing workforce. Partly this was due to high SEN training requirements and the resultant slow rise in SEN pupil numbers.
By September 1958 there were only 9,500 full-time SENs in hospitals, less than in 1949, and most of those had got onto the Roll
through experience, not assessment.[33]
The 1950s and 1960s were marked by further attempts to square
the circle of shortage versus high educational standards. The GNC
focused on selection policies while RCN continued to develop elite
educational programmes – for example, establishing (with HE Colleges) a Sister Tutor Diploma in 1947 (expanded to two years in
1952); this remained the key qualification until 1982.[34] However,
neither institution faced the fundamental flaw: 'the traditional structures of nursing' were at odds with the 'changing roles of women
in the wider society'.[35] Student nurses remained a source of cheap,
moderately skilled hospital labour – an unattractive career choice
for women in a broadening labour market. Abel-Smith concluded
that shortages were caused by the educationalists' naive and counter-
productive rush to professionalize. They were so terrified of further
diluting their definition of the professional nurse that they made it
too exclusive, while still claiming that all (even basic) nursing should
be done only by registered or enrolled practitioners. The reality was
that, in the absence of sufficient numbers of registered and enrolled
nurses, employers were forced to hire less qualified staff. The *Nursing
Mirror* commented in 1955 that it was time to acknowledge that the
logic of professionalization meant an intra-professional hierarchy:

> The plain truth is that the vital qualifications for nursing – basic
> nursing – are personal qualities – compassion, devotion, and com-
> mon sense, however much the highly skilled and highly trained brain
> is demanded for … more complicated … medical and surgical tech-
> niques and … administrative … management. Let us … keep … highly
> trained and skilled nurses for … work requiring special qualifications,
> and let us recognize invaluable and sterling qualities which many
> people, who are not SRN, or even SEAN [State Enrolled Assistant
> Nurse] … bring to the service of the patient …. To recognize the var-
> ious skills, to allocate the various duties and not to seek to restrict the
> whole expanding field of nursing to a single type of worker is not
> necessarily lowering nursing standards.[36]

The logic of a hierarchy of nursing grades performing different tasks
with different skill levels, increasingly implicit in the actual division
of nursing labour in the health-care system, was becoming generally

accepted by nurse leaders by the mid-1950s. It was no longer realistic to insist on a professionalizing strategy that stressed professional unity; there were different types of nurse, even within the hospital. Additionally, with the majority of nurses neither registered or enrolled, and thus not RCN-represented, health unions annexed large swathes, further weakening professionalizers' visions of one, unified profession.

Indeed the old vocationalist versus professionalizer dispute did not go away either, but became a series of questions about professional identity. Did the more specialized nursing grades risk losing touch with the core values and skills of basic human care? Were these values and skills central to the professional identity of *all* nurses, or were technical, scientific skills more relevant to the professional identity of some nurses? Was the growth in specialized nursing redefining care?[37] Nursing became increasingly ideologically polarized around this practice/theory (heart/mind) axis. While educationalist nurse leaders advocated programmes which raised selection and educational standards, and built academic links, the years of open professional access had exacerbated anti-intellectual tendencies amongst traditional vocationalists.

However, for the state and the hospital employers, the student nurse was still just a pair of hands. In 1952, the GNC attempted to re-impose the minimum entry requirement (at 2 O levels), but once again the Ministry backed the hospital authorities' position: student status risked jeopardizing the hospital service. As one hospital management committee put it:

> For so long as 75 per cent of nursing work in the ward is undertaken by nurses in training, and . . . the major part of their time is spent on giving service to the hospital, as distinct from receiving tuition, the real status of the nurse in training is something between that of an apprentice and one serving articles, and not that of student.[38]

A reality-check on nurse education quality was provided by the Nuffield (Goddard) Report of 1953. Wood had wanted to build from the ground up by asking what the nurse's role was, but no quantitative data existed. H. A. Goddard, a management consultant, conducted the first time-and-motion audit of nursing work. He found that formal instruction per week varied from eleven hours to seven minutes; no sister tutor even entered a training school ward during the period of the study; busy ward sisters prioritized patient care over teaching (the exact opposite of the position in medicine); and student nurses were left in charge of wards 22 per cent of the time. Student status was nominal. Additionally, nurse tutors were marginalized in training schools still dominated by matron heads of nursing services.[39]

RCN's response, *Observations and Objectives,* committed the College to developing new cadres of elite leaders in management, teaching and research.[40] By the 1950s, nurse leaders had finally, though reluctantly, embraced a tripartite division of labour on the wards: auxiliaries for domestic work, SENs (with beefed-up training and status) for basic and SRNs for technical nursing, with a super-elite going onto further (university) training as the new educational and managerial leaders.[41] *Observations* specifically committed RCN to nursing degrees, though, as Education Director Mick Carpenter clarified, not for all nurses. While Carpenter stressed RCN's ongoing commitment to the vocational ethos ('the true nursing qualities of practical skill, human understanding, and the all-important sense of vocation'), degrees were a lure for 'bringing into the profession more trained minds with a broad outlook' – those who found nurse training too basic. Such new nurses could be built into an elite cadre of nurses, with higher career paths in 'each branch of nursing for example, clinical, administrative, teaching'.[42]

Such plans synchronized with the epidemiological shift from infectious to the modern chronic diseases (cancer, heart disease and stroke) and the teamwork necessitated by increasingly high-technology scientific medicine. NHS structures and culture also played a role in nurturing the development of medical specialties, which needed new forms of nursing. Spaces also opened up for nurses to take on tasks relinquished by doctors; as doctors became increasingly super-specialized, nurses became specialized in new areas. As well as the three traditional divisions of Adult, Child and Mental Health, there had been specialist nurses (e.g. anaesthetics, infectious diseases, tuberculosis, mental and physical disability) from the late nineteenth century, again shadowing the development of medical and surgical specialties and service provision. And there had also been discrete areas of nursing practice with their specialized knowledge and qualifications (e.g. public health nursing had morphed into infant, school, industrial and tuberculosis nursing). But, beginning in the 1950s, as the rate of medical advance quickened, discrete bodies of nursing knowledge and practice developed around, for example, cardiac care, intensive care, geriatrics and haemodialysis. A useful index is number and range of RCN specialist forums: there were 5 in 1975, 7 in 1976 and 22 in 1982. By 1990 there were 65.[43] Nurse specialization, however, still entailed subservience to the medical paradigm, and this was soon reflected in research that sought to justify and expand specialist roles in both theoretical/technical and managerial spheres. However, specialization rested on the firm establishment of nursing knowledge as a discrete advanced subject for which extended special study (not just practical experience) was needed.

The Platt Report, *A Reform of Nursing Education*, published in 1964, proposed key measures now widely accepted within nursing – the service nexus must be broken:

> *The student nurse should be a student in fact and not in name only* . . . the service . . . she gives must be governed by . . . educational needs . . . . Schools of nursing would be set up . . . outside the hospitals, making use of the hospitals for training . . . like medical students attending university and gaining experience in hospital . . . . University degrees in nursing should be established.[44]

Since society, medicine and patients' expectations had changed, in order to end the shortage of nurses, nursing now had to change too. Unfortunately, many doctors' attitudes had not changed; over-education was unnecessary and risked forfeiting British nurses' characteristic experience-rooted expert knowledge of the practical caring arts:

> what the hospital doctor usually needs is not another colleague with whom to discuss the complexities of acid–base balance. He wants as many intelligent, well-trained nurses as can be found, to look after the needs of the patient. There is certainly a place for a few university-trained nurses . . . but . . . only a few, and they must have as much practical experience as those admirable . . . sisters in . . . teaching hospitals . . . . Most girls who want to be nurses want to be just that – they do not want to be Bachelors of Science, and most girls who want to be Bachelors of Science do not want to be nurses.[45]

Surprisingly, the GNC also rejected Platt; confident that its own measures (new entry requirements, a new syllabus, the recruitment of more tutors and the encouragement of experimental training schemes) would suffice. The Minister of Health agreed with the RCN: that there should be more registered nurses on the wards, but for their 'experienced judgement' rather than for their 'technical skill'.[46] The state/medicine compact still denied nursing the status of a discrete technical knowledge, but nursing soon challenged exactly this *sancta sanctorum*.

Although of little contemporaneous impact, Platt set nursing's educational agenda for 40 years. By 1968 there were already nursing schools offering university-linked courses: the first nursing degree was established in 1960 at the University of Edinburgh, Manchester, followed in 1969 and the polytechnics were close behind (e.g. London's City in 1968, Leeds, Newcastle and South Bank in 1974).[47] However, these accounted for few registrations; most nursing students remained, for now, effectively apprentices.

1950–86: Obstacles to Professionalization

While educationalists fought to convince doctors and state that nursing was a technical expertise with its own knowledge base, existing professional status and identity were threatened by the increasing numbers of men coming into general nursing from the late 1960s. Long present, and dominant in psychiatric nursing since the very first asylums, male nurses had been actively recruited during the acute shortages of the 1930s as the hospital sector expanded and alternative careers opened up for women. Men were admitted to the general Register in 1949 as part of the Nursing Registration Act's attempt to bring in more nurses. Men made up 16 per cent of the workforce by 1950, although this fell back to 11 per cent by 1972, over a period when the NHS workforce had doubled in size. They remained at around 10 per cent of the workforce, although they were more likely to get promotion into the top two senior grades, and by the 1990s enjoyed a disproportionate presence in senior nursing administration and management posts.[48] Male nurses were also more likely to join and take a lead in the radical left-wing politics of trade unionism that polarized British society, including nursing, in the 1970s and 1980s.

The attempt to present a unified professional image also increasingly alienated the less technically specialized district nurses, who felt undervalued and ignored by general hospital nurses. District nurses wanted recognition of their different educational needs and representation on the RCN Council. They finally achieved this in 1971 via their own section, after threatening to leave the College.[49]

Also perceived as pulling at the threads of professionalization was the increasing recruitment of nurses of overseas origin. Like the male nurse, the black nurse further undermined the existing model of unified professional identity based on the nurse as an educated, middle-class (white) woman. Overseas recruitment for all types of nursing and support staff was pursued vigorously from the mid-1940s by the Health and Labour Departments in the former colonies (especially the Caribbean and Africa) to combat the nursing shortage. In 1968, there were over 17,000 overseas nurses training in Britain;[50] by 1971, overseas student nurses and midwives made up 12 per cent of the total, and of these 66 per cent were Afro-Caribbean.[51] Like South Asian doctors, the state used them as cheap labour in lower grades to prop-up the health service in times of staff shortage.[52] They came to train as general SRNs and ended up as SENs in physically and emotionally draining 'Cinderella' specialties like geriatrics or mental disability. Neither grade nor specialty was of any use when they returned home, so many stayed. At the same time, it was claimed – somewhat disingenuously – that this was a form of overseas development aid.[53] However, this expansion of the lower nursing grades also again raised the spectre of de-professionalization. Although they were helping to staff the NHS, overseas nurses were seen as a problem; bad for professional image and status. Echoing the GMC's 1970s position on overseas doctors, the RCN argued, without any evidence, that Commonwealth nurses were dumbing-down the profession and that over-reliance on them kept pay and conditions low for all.[54] In fact, Commonwealth student nurses did better in their professional examinations than those from other countries.[55]

It was not surprising that professional tensions aroused by black nurses and the educational aspersions they generated were first publicly expressed in evidence to Briggs. The committee, charged with reviewing all nursing roles and education in a soon-to-be reorganized NHS, became dominated by educational interests and embodied the long-standing educationalist manifesto. However, only Briggs's suggested regulatory structure – that there should be a unitary statutory pre/post-registration regulatory body for the whole of the United Kingdom – was incorporated into the 1978 Nurses, Midwives and Health Visitors Act, which established the United Kingdom Central Council.[56]

Briggs did confirm the contention that nursing was not an occupational workforce, but a profession with an expert knowledge base 'separate from but equal to the medical profession'.[57] Nursing was soon to take the logical professionalizing step and argue the case for autonomous practice. This was done by the development of nursing research, which set out to build a robust evidence base to support professional claims to unique and discrete expertise in the theory and practice of nursing, via educational and managerial routes. Largely separate epistemologies and methodologies of nursing were developed for each of these versions of professionalization: the educated nurse and the nurse as manager.

1950–86: Professionalization and the Development of Nursing Research

The failings of nursing education identified by the Nuffield Report (in particular, the limited attention paid to the learning needs of student nurses, evident in the limited teaching they received while in practice, and the use of students to take charge of wards) also catalyzed the development of research on nursing roles and tasks.[58] University links began to develop. In 1953 Edinburgh University established (with a Boots grant) the first nursing fellowship. In 1958, RCN appointed Marjorie Simpson as Research Officer, and in 1959 the small number of UK nursing researchers came together to form the RCN Research Discussion Group, later the Research Society (1975).[59] The methodology and focus of nursing research was shaped by these early studies of nurse selection and nursing work. It was characterized by 'a pragmatic, theoretical approach, utilising survey methods and quantitative forms of analysis, based in service settings such as hospitals and health authority offices rather than in the academic setting of universities'.[60] In order to take control of the educational agenda, plans were announced in 1960 to publish a dedicated research reports series entitled *RCN Studies in Nursing*, and an advisory research committee was established providing research services.[61]

As Research Officer at the Ministry of Health from 1963, Simpson shaped a state-funded programme to develop the essential infrastructure to enable nursing research to become central to practice. This included practical and theoretical groundwork of various kinds: firstly, the establishment of a research fellowship scheme from 1967 providing research training for nurses taking higher degrees; secondly, the recruitment of regional nursing liaison officers to advise on research; and thirdly, the establishment of five nursing research units (e.g. at the RCN to develop methods for measuring nursing care quality, and at the GNC to evaluate experimental education programmes). Finally, research fora were launched: the *Index of Nursing Research* (1976) and the journal *Nursing Research Abstracts* (1978); and joint funding of the *RCN Research Monographs* series.

The most influential outcome was the MH/DHSS-funded RCN 1967–74 study of nursing care quality indicators led by Jean McFarlane, which resulted in her *The Proper Study of the Nurse* (1970) and Ursula Inman's *Towards a Theory of Nursing Care* (1975). The nine, discrete, empirical studies were designed to show how 'the research methods of a wide range of disciplines can be applied to nursing problems' to determine concrete, quantifiable methods of 'measuring the effectiveness of nursing care'.[62] They sought to justify nursing as an independent academic study with its own 'principles and laws; it must be neither lesser medicine nor a phase of social work, but valuable in itself'.[63]

These studies seeded the future principles and practice of UK nursing research in four key ways. Firstly, the study of nursing practice, the nursing models developed and especially the standards of care theme became central to research into the 1990s. Secondly, the project provided evidence for the claim of a strong link between quality of care and nurse staffing levels. Thirdly, the studies firmly established the principles that all nurses needed to ground their practice in research, that teaching should also be research-based and that, consequently, some nurses needed to specialize to produce that research. The project itself also began to train up those researchers: research assistants became the first professors of nursing in, and heads of, the new academic nursing departments.[64] Underlining the new centrality of research to the RCN educationalist strategy, McFarlane left the project in 1968 to become RCN Education Director. In 1974 she became the holder of the first Chair of Nursing in an English university, at Manchester.

In the concluding monograph of the RCN research series, however, Inman charted a new course. The role of nursing research was 'to establish a unique body of nursing knowledge … thereby strengthening nurses' professionalism'. Whereas nursing research's previous nascent directions were too focused at the workplace level of pay, conditions and staffing, Inman argued that 'the proper study of the nurse' is not the nurse, but *nursing*: not the conditions of work but its theory and practice.[65] Moreover, she put forward a new definition of nursing care. Nursing was almost infinitely heterogeneous, and the meaning of care changed over time: 'while we are busy describing the latest type of care it is already changing'.[66] Characterizing all the essential elements of nursing as a discrete disciplinary entity was impossible. Instead Inman subordinated it to medical knowledge. Meanings and quality of nursing care should be measured by how far they met *medically* defined patient needs: 'for the patients' therapeutic needs are normative needs in this context and as nurses we are bound to carry out medically prescribed care.[67] Basic and psychological needs should also be provided, and worked out by the nurse, but these categories were severely delimited to include only general care needs and minimization of patient anxiety.[68]

This was a much stronger formulation than Virginia Henderson's influential 1958 patient needs-based definition, which first made the case for nursing knowledge as specialized and scientific.[69] Inman now defined the 'proper' nature and scope of nursing work more broadly and specifically as incorporating control of the *whole* healing environment. This was a claim that nursing expertise was fundamentally also managerial: the quality of nursing care depended on the 'conceptual or planning skill of the sister or charge nurse' and her degree of control of a range of relevant variables – the physical 'layout and facilities', staffing levels (including nursing/support staff skill and grade-mix), 'the allocation and supervision of work', information and its communication and 'the skill level of training of nursing staff'.[70] The strategic payoff from this avowal of subservience to medicine was nurse control of whole ward environments; as Inman argued: 'I do not believe that the problems of measuring the quality of nursing care will ever be solved by examining only specific areas of nursing care. The patient admitted to a hospital ward experiences a total system of nursing care.'[71] Inman was adding research authority to the traditional call for the unity of hospital nursing activities, at a time when nurses' power in the control of nursing policy at all levels was reaching a temporary apogee. This was the beginning of a new claim to professional monopoly over the specialized content and organization of integrated holistic care, which would soon be used to push for full autonomy, but was ultimately to fall foul of changing political and NHS cultures.

In a radical shift in professionalization strategy, Inman also introduced the idea of nursing as a *process*: an efficient structure for nursing work that embodied research-derived best practice at every step. The nursing process[72] was a set of programmatic tasks, fundamental to healing, that complemented medicine, but could only be performed by a trained nurse. It again underlined that nursing had a unique and robust way of applying scientific approaches to both the management and the (increasingly) technical content of nursing work. It was thus an argument for professional, clinical autonomy that stressed both managerial and educational aspects of the new nursing.

The nursing process became central to nursing discourses very quickly. It was first discussed among nurses in 1973. By 1975 the first articles about it had been published, and by 1977 it was part of general nursing's pre-registration curriculum, with the first British book following in 1979. In the United Kingdom, the nursing process was focused on improving care quality and nurse job satisfaction,[73] but, at the same time, it embodied the first definitive professional autonomy claim. First promulgated by Manchester University's Department of Nursing, the nursing process used Henderson's concept of patient-centred care[74] to argue for discrete therapeutic roles for nursing, thus removing its subservience to medicine. Each patient was systematically assessed: a nursing history was taken, nursing needs identified, the nursing methods necessary to meet these needs were then planned and results of delivery nurse-assessed. Nursing was a therapy in its own right, with its own distinctive, holistic, knowledge-base, staffing mix/levels and organization necessary for healing; it was not subordinate but complementary to medicine.[75]

The research-supported nursing process, as a rationale for professional autonomy, led to innovations such as Nurse Development Units, primary nursing and nurse practitioners.[76] Research was integrated into the pre-registration curriculum by the late 1980s, but the fact that the Department of Health had to reemphasize the need for all nurses to become research-literate as late as 1993 does raise the question of how far nursing practice had become evidence-based by then.[77] Also, old interests obstructed the path. The turn towards individual nurse autonomy in the educationalists' professional strategy occurred just as the Conservative government looked to cut health budgets via close auditing of all NHS activities to ensure cost-effectiveness. By the late 1980s, nursing and midwifery accounted for around 47 per cent of the entire NHS pay spend, and this figure was increasing. In 1991, the Audit Commission argued nursing's ward establishments and skill-mix were *ad hoc* and illogical, not based on a fundamental definition of nursing. Ironically, the nursing process facilitated nursing audit; it easily became a managerial tool – an atomistic analysis and justification for every nursing activity.[78]

1986–2000: Professional Maturity, Education and Management

The first element of the new educational strategy was establishing the research culture; its second was the reorientation towards higher education and proper student status for trainees. Project 2000 (P2000) dominated the educational agenda into the twenty-first century. In 1986 UKCC produced *Project 2000: A New Preparation for Practice*, which recommended a three-year diploma (or four-year degree) taught at nursing schools, increasingly based in higher education, with curricula containing academic subjects. New courses would share a common foundation course followed by specialized training; enrolled nurse training would end; all nurse teachers should have degrees; and all student nurses would be supernumerary on hospital wards, contributing minimally to service. However, students then accounted for one quarter of the NHS labour force and provided three quarters of hospital ward direct care. It was thus unsurprising when, in 1988, the government, while agreeing to educational reform, accepted only a diluted version of P2000 in which students gave 20 per cent of their total time to ward work; enrolled nurse training continued for five years; and phasing out was linked to a new junior grade of health–care support worker, covering basic care. Arguably, the government had only accepted moving nurse education to higher education because it fitted with imminent plans to reorganize the NHS around trusts, rather than area health authorities: once again nursing's priorities were not a key factor in change. Moreover, in accepting this compromise, nursing committed itself to a much smaller future elite of trained nurses.[79]

P2000 aimed to produce a new type of nurse – the 'knowledgeable doer' – who could implement the holistic nursing process with her ability to 'marshal information, to make an assessment of need, devise a plan of care and implement, monitor and evaluate it'.[80] However, the new academic curricula fragmented the claim to a unique nursing expertise by incorporating increased amounts of sociological, psychological and physical science, and thus, arguably, alienating knowledge from practice.[81]

Nurse educators themselves became increasingly concerned that academic courses did not reflect practical ward realities. By 1991, the ratio of qualified to unqualified hospital nursing staff had dropped from 61:23 to 58:28[82] and continued falling, while numbers of less qualified staff increased, as government-funded replacements covered only half the student nurses moving off ward into universities; ward nursing's skill mix became highly contentious.

But it was nurse education that suffered a backlash from nurses as 'rejection of the academic content of nurse education became a fundamental problem in the implementation of Project 2000'.[83] There was still no professional consensus that 'theory would enhance practice and not diminish clinical skills', as the new model nurses failed to meet the high expectations of clinical confidence fundamental to P2000.[84] Many nurses saw degrees as a professional necessity, others felt strongly that 'nursing is a practical hands-on' activity: academic focus devalued the practical art of caring.[85] In 1999, the UKCC proposed that a new practical competency-based model should be integrated into training.[86]

Educationalists responded with two robust defences of P2000's academicization agenda: *Making a Difference* (DoH, 1999) and *Fitness for Practice* (UKCC, 1999), arguing that the problem was not too much, but too little academic content. Educational goals had been weakened by NHS and higher education changes; even closer university links were needed in a revised curriculum that would deliver all necessary modern practice skills.[87] But closer academic links risked a further destabilization of professional identity: academics could claim that their disciplines, and not 'nursing', were the core skills being taught. In some universities nursing was tolerated as a revenue-generating junior partner, despised by many theory-laden academics for its low-status practice connotations and coveted by others as a territory ripe for colonization.[88]

In spite of increased academicization, nursing ended the century facing the same constraints on its educational professionalization strategy that it faced in 1920: an uncertain professional identity caught between the division of medical labour and the rationed funds and politicized priorities of the health-care delivery system. If anything, the professional progress achieved (in terms of pay and conditions and professional status[89]) sharpened these constraints: nurses were now more of a threat and an expensive irritation, especially since the advent of the culture of micro-level health-care auditing for effectiveness and efficiency. Under post-1979 governments, nursing expertise was systematically devalued by a bureaucratization process which increasingly imported business management methods into health-care delivery. Some groups of nurses tried to meet this challenge head-on by developing a new professional version of the nurse as manager, building on Nightingale's organizational tradition, and the administrative authority of traditional matrons and re-equipping it with evolving managerial discourses. Just as nursing research had fleshed out the evidence base supporting nursing's claim to authority as a science, so it now provided organizational models to deliver measurable doses of optimum care. However, although mangerialism made some gains, ultimately, like educationalism, it left nurses at the mercy of other professional groups whose health-care expertise became more highly socially recognized and valued.

The idea of the nurse as manager is traced back by its adherents to the organizational philosophy of Nightingale. Post-Nightingale hospital matrons enjoyed wide-ranging managerial powers as part of their unified authority. Its gradual erosion from 1948 made nurses super-watchful. The Nuffield Report's recommendation of total, holistic care was interpreted by RCN as removing administrative roles: perceived as part of the indivisible whole of nursing and directly related to patient well-being. Indeed, in the 1960s, as part of the return to holistic nursing campaign, 'managerialist discourse was actually deployed as a vehicle of professional advancement by the nursing leadership'.[90] Some nurses claimed managerial role equality with administrators and RCN began managerial training courses to develop managerial leaders. In 1964 it published *Administering the Hospital Nursing Services* which posited higher nurse career structures in administration, education and clinical nursing. Currently, it was argued, in contrast to medicine, nursing's clinical ladder ended at ward sister, an increasingly arduous post. Ambitious nurses must then divert into administration, which itself lacked systematic structure and effective nurse representation at policy level. In 1967, the Ministry of Health succumbed to such pressure and appointed Brian Salmon, chairman of Lyons catering group, to advise on the structure and management of hospital nursing. The Salmon Report[91] attempted to introduce a modern line-management structure into the nursing service, and to synchronize with the existing NHS organization. It finally removed the matrons' unified power, replacing it with three new tiers of nursing management: first-line ward managers (staff nurses and ward sisters) undertaking task allocation; middle-managers (Nursing Officers) executing resource planning and purchasing – an opportunity for experienced clinical practitioners to feed in expertise; and finally top-management (new Chief Nursing Officers at hospital-group level, supported by specialty principal nursing officers) to transmit national nursing policy to hospital management committees.

However government budgets were tight in 1966–7 and so pilot-scheme roll-outs were rushed and underfunded. Nurses also received either no managerial training or inappropriate managerial training for new posts. Few understood the intended operations of new structures. Moreover, Nursing Officers' clinical influence was resisted by ward sisters and consultants, and the post etiolated. Salmon did, however, prepare nurse managers for the new roles they would have after the 1974 reorganization. The new Regional-Area-District organization was implemented by management teams of doctors, nurses, administrators and finance officers at each level with responsibilities organized by function. The UK Chief Nursing Officer managed all nursing staff and the whole nursing budget. This professional, consensus management gave nursing immense, unprecedented power. Nurses now had a voice at every level of management and, because of relative workforce size, control of a huge portion of NHS funds. Local Chief Nursing Officers were able to develop supportive administrative teams to manage staffing issues, clinical issues and nurse education.

In addition, as we saw above, nursing research and the nursing process created an evidence base in the 1960s and 1970s to support the idea of the nurse as scientific manager (as well as scientific practitioner), uniquely skilled in rational decision-making processes and in the relationship between skill-mix and the delivery of measurably high-quality care. In fact discourses of quantitative measures of 'effectiveness and outcomes' 'colonized'[92] the way that the profession was framed in the 1980s and 1990s by certain groups of nurses advancing the nurse as the best type of manager.[93] Nurse academic Michael Traynor observed in 1999 that:

> One aim ... of professional development is the nurse who can articulate her objectives, demonstrate and measure her impact using particular criteria ... can manage a team of lesser skilled workers, and who is constantly questioning whether the same effect can be achieved more efficiently.[94]

Many nurses feared that the new managerial culture was anathema to the characteristic core of nursing's professional identity: the concept of holistic care. However, some nursing research tackled this controversial issue head on by attempting translations that would express holism in the dominant new language of general management. The debate about task versus patient allocation was partly an attempt to put forward a form of nursing management which was compatible with a strongly patient-centred focus.[95] Attempts were made to capture tacit knowledge about good practice and optimum patient-experience in the new managerial language; a flood of books and articles were published on measuring the quality of care.[96] By the century's end, this had become a deluge, as generating effectiveness and efficiency data for nursing's evidence base became a key professional requirement.

The post-Salmon autonomy, however, was short-lived as the incoming Conservative governments (1979–92) viewed consensus as a recipe for administrative inertia and, worse, inefficiency and overspending. The new managerialism championed the methods of late twentieth-century corporate capitalism: the perpetual, rigorous, qualitative and quantitative analysis of products, processes and services to identify cost-efficiency savings, implemented through rationalization. The 1983 Griffiths report's famous comment that Nightingale wouldn't find anybody in charge in the NHS was part of ideological attacks on weaker professions. There were managers, but not the right sort: general business management was now the required expertise, not nursing management.[97] Government so liked this ideology that every level was given general managers, and nursing officers lost control of nursing: the national Chief Nursing Officer was no longer on the new Supervisory Board; local Chief Nursing Officers lost control of nursing budgets, nursing workforce issues and nursing education; even ward sisters were now responsible to general business managers. Management by professionals had been replaced by professional management.

Conclusion

In the period from 1920 to 2000, nursing was constructed by two contingent professionalizing discourses. Educationalists attempted to emulate medicine's professional trajectory towards high-status graduate entry, while managerialists tried to re-route the vocationalists' authority through the culture of private sector general management. Fortified by the increasing dominance of the hospital as the locus of care, these discourses were complicated by interplays of class, gender and ethnicity, and by the emergence of nursing specialties. Both the educationalists and the managerialists hoped to transform the rank-and-file, and to create new elite career pathways into a super policy-elite. However, both failed, constrained by nursing's subordinate position to medicine, and by the medical profession's mutually reinforcing relations with the state, embedded in the very structure of the NHS. Moreover, these attempts at professionalization were self-defeating: they alienated nurse leaders from the grass roots and left an even more divided occupational group.

As Baly argued, 'nursing' is shaped by social change.[98] By the same token, the concept of the nursing 'profession' has been defined in different ways over time by different groups of nursing leaders, and this has affected the content of nurse education and research.[99] Most recently, academic and economic rationalist discourses have infected nursing, as nurse leaders sought to absorb the socio-cultural authority of science and rational management.[100] However, though nurse leaders have tried to express the enduring humanistic core values of nursing in the new discourses, many nurses have perceived a deep antipathy and incompatibility between those values and such discourses. These worries have partly fuelled the anti-intellectualist backlash among nurses (and the wider public) against the move to nursing as an academic subject, a conservative stance which ever-reactionary medical professional interests have been keen to endorse:

> This is why Granny has bedsores. This is why there are no nurses on the wards .... These nurses are all 'graduates' now. They have their BSc (Bedpan) from the University of Formerpoly and have thus become too important to carry out basic nursing care. Instead, they are busy sitting in offices, endlessly filling in forms and ticking boxes to prove that patient care has never been better.[101]

How can nursing find a robust professional identity when pulled in all directions by such titanic social interests? A way out of this potentially mortal nexus has recently been suggested by Nursing Professor Davina Allen. There has been, she argued, a:

> mismatch between real life nursing work and the profession's occupational mandate with its emphasis on emotionally intimate therapeutic relationships with patients. Not only does this produce exaggerated expectations of *practice*, it fails to provide nurses with a knowledge base and a language with which to articulate what it is they do in *practice*.

Nursing's professional, ideological, epistemological and educational focus should not be the nurse, the patient, nor nurs-*ing*, but the entire health-care system. This is 'more effective at mitigating ... [its] objectifying tendencies ... than time spent at the bedside', and will deliver 'a more sustainable professional future'.[102] The nurse should be the patient's 'advocate', promoting and protecting their vulnerable interests.[103]

This recalls Pearce's 1937 definition of nurses as interpreter/integrator of the bewildering alien world of the hospital, with its wide range of clinical contacts, to frightened patients.[104] It is a new way of expressing the human perspective central to nursing that returns the focus to the role of the individual nurse and her relationship with the individual patient.[105] Although this unique skill of subjective connection in an objectifying environment has been constrained by medical and state interests, and has often seemed eclipsed as nurses struggled to express it in the professionalizing languages of educationalists and managerialists, it always returns as the enduring basis of nursing's contribution: the light that never goes out.

Notes

1. C. Nottingham, 'The Rise of the Insecure Professionals', *International Review of Social History*, 52:4 (2007) 464, 460.
2. R. White, 'Political Regulators in British Nursing', in R. White (ed.), *Political Issues in Nursing 1* (Chichester: John Wiley, 1986); R. White, 'From Matron to Manager', in R. White (ed.), *Political Issues in Nursing 2* (Chichester: John Wiley, 1986).
3. C. Davies, *Gender and the Professional Predicament in Nursing* (Buckingham: Open University Press, 1995). See also: A.Witz, *Professions and Patriarchy* (London: Routledge, 1992); A.M. Rafferty, *The Politics of Nursing Knowledge* (London: Routledge, 1996).
4. R. Dingwall, A.M. Rafferty and C. Webster, *An Introduction to the Social History of Nursing* (London: Routledge, 1988) p. 228.
5. M. Carpenter, 'The Subordination of Nurses in Healthcare: Towards a Social Divisions Approach', in W. Riska and K. Wegar (eds), *Gender, Work and Medicine* (London: Sage, 1993) pp. 95–130.
6. E. Pearce, *General Textbook of Nursing* (London: Faber, 1937) p. 4.
7. *Idem*, 17th edn (London: Faber, 1967) p. 21.
8. *Idem*, 20th edn (London: Faber, 1980) p. xvii.
9. K. Melia, *Learning and Working* (London: Tavistock, 1987).
10. H. Sweet and R. Dougall, *Community Nursing and Primary Healthcare in Twentieth Century Britain* (Abingdon: Routledge, 2008) p. 210.
11. B. Abel-Smith, *A History of the Nursing Profession* (London: Heinemann, 1961) pp. 99–113.
12. Abel-Smith, *History*, p. 154.
13. Abel-Smith, *History*, pp. 118–19.
14. Abel-Smith, *History*, pp. 148–75; Dingwall, Rafferty and Webster, *Introduction*, pp. 77–97; J. Salvage, *The Politics of Nursing* (London: Heinemann, 1985) pp. 95–101.
15. 'Making the Future Nurse', *Nursing Times* (7 May 1921) 498, cited in Rafferty, *Politics*, p. 118.
16. Rafferty, *Politics*.
17. S. McGann, A. Crowther and R. Dougall, *A History of the Royal College of Nursing* (Manchester: Manchester University Press, 2009) p. 50.

18. G. Rivett, *National Health Service History*, http://nhshistory.com, accessed 22 February 2011.
19. M. Green, 'Nursing Education', in M. Baly (ed.), *Nursing and Social Change*, 3rd edn (London: Routledge, 1995) pp. 295–310.
20. Abel-Smith, *History*, pp. 151–5.
21. J. Hallam, *Nursing the Image: Media, Culture and Professional Identity* (London, Routledge, 2000) p. 87.
22. Abel-Smith, *History*, p. 143; Dingwall, Rafferty and Webster, *Introduction*, pp. 126–30.
23. See Abel-Smith, *History*, pp. 130–90; Baly, *Nursing*, pp.157–79; Dingwall, Rafferty and Webster, *Introduction*, pp. 98–122; Rafferty, *Politics*, pp. 113–81; McGann, Crowther and Dougall, *History*, pp. 86–159.
24. R. White, *The Effects of the National Health Service on the Nursing Profession* (London: King's Fund, 1985) pp. 27–9.
25. White, *Effects*, p. 40.
26. Abel-Smith, *History*, p.188.
27. RCN Nursing Reconstruction Committee, *Minutes* (20 January 1942) 57, cited in Rafferty, *Politics*, p. 171.
28. Dingwall, Rafferty and Webster, *Introduction*. pp. 118–19.
29. Hallam, *Nursing*, p. 95.
30. Hallam, *Nursing*; White, 'Political Regulators'; White, 'From Matron'.
31. White, *Effects*, pp. 52–88; Baly, *Nursing*, pp. 197–9, 277–80.
32. Abel-Smith, *History*, pp. 211–12.
33. Abel-Smith, *History*, pp. 234–5.
34. Green, 'Nursing Education', pp. 296–7.
35. Dingwall, Rafferty and Webster, *Introduction*, p. 119.
36. 'Editorial', *Nursing Mirror* (10 June 1955) 720, cited by Abel-Smith, *History*, p. 237.
37. J. Hallam, 'Ethical Lives in the Early Nineteenth Century: Nursing and a History of Caring', in B. Mortimer and S. McGann (eds), *New Directions in the History of Nursing* (Abingdon: Routledge, 2005) pp. 22–39.
38. Luton and Hitchin Hospital Management Committee, 'Some Current Problems of Nurse Training, 10 June 1953', cited in McGann, Crowther and Dougall, *History,* pp. 185–6.
39. McGann, Crowther and Dougall, *History*, pp. 186; J. Brooks, ' "Women In-between": The Ambiguous Position of the Sister Tutor', *Nurse Education Today*, 27 (2007) 169–75.
40. Rivett, *National Health Service History*.
41. McGann, Crowther and Dougall, *History*, pp. 164–76.
42. M. Carpenter, 'Degrees in Nursing', *British Medical Journal* (29 December 1956) 1546.
43. McGann, Crowther and Dougall, *History*, pp. 226–7.

44. R. Girdwood, 'Some Problems of Nursing Today', *British Medical Journal* (4 June 1966) 1411–13. My emphasis.
45. Girdwood, 'Some Problems'.
46. McGann, Crowther and Dougall, *History*, pp. 215–22.
47. Green, 'Nursing Education', p. 302.
48. C. Mackintosh, 'A Historical Study of Men in Nursing', *Journal of Advanced Nursing*, 26 (1997) 232–6; Hallam, *Nursing*, pp. 112–17.
49. Dingwall, Rafferty and Webster, *Introduction*, pp. 173–203; McGann, Crowther and Dougall, *History*, pp. 263–4.
50. Hallam (2000), *Nursing*, pp. 117–24.
51. E. Jones and S. Snow, *Against the Odds* (Manchester: Manchester Primary Care Trust, 2010) p. 19.
52. See A. Hull and S. Bhattacharya, 'Health Service Sepoys? The Role of South Asian Doctors in the NHS, c.1944–80', Institucio Mila I Fontanals, *History of Science Working Papers* 1 (2006) 1–18.
53. Hallam, *Nursing*, p. 119.
54. RCN Evidence to the Committee on Nursing (London: RCN, 1971), cited in Hallam, *Nursing*, p. 120.
55. Hallam, *Nursing*, p. 120; Jones and Snow, *Against the Odds*, pp. 8–10; 50–69.
56. Dingwall, Rafferty and Webster, *Introduction*, pp. 206–10.
57. Dingwall, Rafferty and Webster, *Introduction*, p. 209
58. Green, 'Nursing Education', p. 313.
59. McGann, Crowther and Dougall, *History*, p. 175.
60. Green, 'Nurse Education', p. 313.
61. 'History of the Research Society', rcn.org.uk/development/research anddevelopment/rs/history, accessed 12 April 2011; White, *Effects*, pp. 216–30.
62. U. Inman, *Towards a Theory of Nursing Care: An Account of the RCN/DHSS Research Project 'The Study of Nursing Care'* (London: RCN, 1975) p. 80.
63. G. Carter, 'Collegiate Education for Nursing', *Nursing Times* (15 August 1953) 812–13.
64. Inman, *Towards*, p. 80.
65. Inman, *Towards*, p. 112. My emphasis.
66. Inman, *Towards*, p. 88.
67. Inman, *Towards*, p. 62.
68. Inman, *Towards*, p. 81.
69. White, *Effects*, p. 229.
70. Inman, *Towards*, p. 102.
71. Inman, *Towards*, pp. 102, 111.
72. This was originally an American concept. See I. Orlando, *The Dynamic Nurse-Patient Relationship* (New York: Putnams, 1966).

73. C. De La Cuesta, 'The Nursing Process: From Development to Implementation', *Journal of Advanced Nursing*, 8 (1983) 365–71; Dingwall, Rafferty and Webster, *Introduction*, pp. 213–21; Rivett, *National Health Service History*; B. Salter, *The Politics of Change in the Health Service* (Houndmills: Palgrave Macmillan, 1998), pp. 129–54.

74. UK nursing models followed, rooted in Henderson's approach. Most influential was the Roper–Logan–Tierney human needs model (based on living activities: physiological; psychological, socio-cultural, and politico-economical, and environmental). See N. Roper, W. Logan and A. Tierney, *The Elements of Nursing* (London: Churchill, 1980).

75. C. A. Hale, *Innovations in Nursing Care: A Study of a Change to Patient Centred Care* (London: RCN, 1987).

76. De La Cuesta, 'Nursing Process', p. 139.

77. Department of Health, *Report of the Taskforce on the Strategy for Research in Nursing, Midwifery and Health Visiting* (London: DoH, 1993), cited in P. Moule and M. Goodman, *Nursing Research* (London: Sage, 2009); Salter, *Politics*, p. 135; De La Cuesta, 'Nursing Process'.

78. Salter, *Politics*, pp. 133–43; Dingwall, Rafferty and Webster, *Introduction*, pp. 212–16.

79. Salter, *Politics*, pp. 146–54; Dingwall, Rafferty and Webster, *Introduction*, pp. 221–9; Rivett, *National Health Service History*; McGann, Crowther and Dougall, *History*, pp. 303–5; D. Allen, *The Changing Shape of Nursing Practice* (London: Routledge, 2001), pp. 1–21.

80. UKCC, *Project 2000: The Final Proposals* (London: UKCC, 1987) p. 140.

81. See Melia, *Learning*.

82. D. Allen and P. Lyne, 'How Did We Get There?', in D. Allen and P. Lyne (eds), *Reality of Nursing Research* (London: Routledge, 2006) p. 17.

83. M. Lord, 'Making a Difference', *Nursing Times*, 98:20 (14 May 2002) 38.

84. Lord, 'Making a Difference', p. 38.

85. Readers' Comments, S. Ford, 'All New Nurses Must Have Degrees', *Nursing Times* (12 November 2009).

86. Allen and Lyne, 'How Did We Get There?', p. 17.

87. Lord, 'Making a Difference', p. 38.

88. Allen and Lyne, 'How Did We Get There?', p. 17.

89. C. Hart, *Behind the Mask* (London: Baillière Tindall, 1994).

90. Allen and Lyne, 'How Did We Get There?', p. 14. This section also relies on J Clark, 'Nurses as Managers', in Baly, *Nursing*, pp. 277–94; D. Blenkinsop, 'The Preparation of Nurse Managers', in P. Allan and M. Jolly (eds), *Nursing, Midwifery and Health Visiting* (London: Faber, 1982) pp. 158–65; Rivett, *National Health Service History*; McGann, Crowther and Dougall, *History*; Dingwall, Rafferty and Webster, *Introduction*.

91. *Report of the Committee on Senior Nursing Staff Structure* (London: HMSO, 1966).
92. M. Traynor, *Managerialism and Nursing* (London: Routledge, 1999).
93. M. Walton, *Management and Managing* (London: Lippincott Nursing Series/Harper and Row, 1984).
94. Traynor, *Managerialism*, p. 82.
95. Hale, *Innovations.*
96. Traynor, *Managerialism*; RCN, *Towards Standards* (London: RCN, 1981); A. DiCenso, N. Cullum and D. Cilisk, 'Implementing Evidence-Based Nursing: Some Misconceptions', *Evidence-Based Nursing*, 1:2 (1988) 38–40.
97. *NHS Management Enquiry* DA (83) 38 (1983) DHSS.
98. Baly, *Nursing*, p. xiii.
99. Traynor, *Managerialism*, p. 83.
100. Traynor, *Managerialism*, p. 82.
101. 'Dr. Crippen', 'Only in Our Points-Obsessed System could Nurses Be "Better" than Doctors', *The Guardian* (19 January 2010).
102. D. Allen, 'Re-reading Nursing and Re-writing Practice: Towards an Empirically Based Reformulation of the Nursing Mandate', *Nursing Inquiry*, 11:4 (2004) 271–83.
103. Nursing and Midwifery Council website, http://www.nmc-uk.org/Nurses-and-midwives/Advice-by-topic/A/Advice/Advocacy-and-autonomy/, accessed 12 June 2011.
104. Pearce, *General Textbook of Nursing* (1937), pp. 1–3.
105. See the NMC code (note the very first entreaty) http://www.nmc-uk.org/Nurses-and-midwives/The-code/The-code-in-full/#dignity, accessed 12 June 2011.

PART II

MIDWIFERY 1700–2000

The second part of the book considers the history of midwifery between 1700 and 2000 in three chronological stages. These chapters can be read as standalone chapters or sequentially to provide a chronology of midwifery over the past three centuries. As suggested in the Introduction to Part I of the book, the reader may wish to compare historical developments within midwifery to developments in nursing. A number of similarities and differences can be identified. The following chapters draw particular attention to the specific concerns of midwives and how these changed over the period: the primary focus on childbirth and the influence of cultural attitudes to birth on midwives' work; the scope of midwives' practice and their degree of occupational autonomy; the relationships between female midwives and their male counterparts.

In Chapter 5: *Midwifery, 1700–1800: The Man-Midwife as Competitor,* Helen King describes the situation in the eighteenth century. This was a critical period for midwifery history, when there was growing scientific interest in conception, birth and the reproductive body. Science had begun to dispute the accepted knowledge of traditional childbirth attendants, and as a result the role of the female midwife was challenged by the rise of the man-midwife. King describes the strategies utilized by men-midwives to rise in status, claiming authority over normal as well as difficult births. The position of female midwives deteriorated, although, as King shows, a complex inter-relationship began to develop, as the practice of men-midwives remained dependent on the clinical expertise and skills of female midwives.

Chapter 6: *Midwifery 1800–1920: The Journey to Registration* by Alison Nuttall takes us into the nineteenth century. This was a period of significant change, which saw the transition of British midwifery from that of local women trained informally via apprenticeship to formally trained professionals whose practice was tightly defined and controlled as the result of the 1902 Midwives' Act. Nuttall shows how although enshrining the role of the midwife in UK legislation provided many benefits, this came at a price as the autonomy experienced by midwives earlier in the century was compromised. She draws attention to the influence which doctors exerted on the practice and education of midwives, and the growing tensions between the two occupations, particularly in relation to securing the custom of clients.

In the final chapter in this part, *Midwifery 1920–2000: The Reshaping of a Profession*, Billie Hunter takes us to the end of the twentieth century. Analysing the rapid changes which occurred in midwifery education and practice during this period, Hunter explores how these were influenced by shifts in the conceptualization of childbirth, including understandings of normality and abnormality, nature and science. In particular, Hunter considers how the midwife's role was influenced not only by the pursuit of professional status but also by broader contextual factors, including the effects of the Second World War and the advent of the National Health Service (NHS) and also by shifting public attitudes and political debates related to place of birth and the respective roles of midwife and doctor.

5

Midwifery, 1700–1800: The Man-Midwife as Competitor

Helen King

The eighteenth century was a central period in the history of British midwifery, during which there was widespread interest in the origin of life, the birth process and the social control of the reproductive body.[1] Galenic medicine, based on the ideas of the great second-century AD physician and focused on the four humours, continued to play a very important part in thinking about midwifery; but new ways of seeing the body, drawn from developments based on classification, measurement, mathematics and mechanics, played an increasingly important role. This is not to say that midwifery became 'science'; it is clear that superstitions coexisted with these scientific ideas. For example, it was widely believed that babies born with the caul could not subsequently be drowned or have their houses set on fire.[2] Tales of extraordinary births also convinced large audiences, including medical professionals; most notably, Mary Toft's 1726 claim to have given birth to rabbits as a result of 'maternal impression', the theory that what a woman saw at conception or while pregnant would influence the unborn child.[3] But the new scientific procedures themselves generated superstition. Pierre Dionis thus recommended that, when performing a Caesarean on a dead woman, one should 'put a Gag into her Mouth, to keep it open' because 'the vulgar' think that the child breathes in the womb, and if it is taken out dead then they will blame the surgeon for not keeping the woman's mouth open.[4]

How did the traditional midwife fare, in this world of science and superstition? Her position deteriorated significantly after 1700. For women outside the major towns in particular, the midwife had not only been the main provider of care in childbirth but also traditionally worked in related areas: the disorders of children and conditions affecting women's bodies beyond those associated with giving birth. By 1800, the situation was very different. The cause was the rise of the man-midwife, who had succeeded in claiming control over the management not just of difficult births but also of normal labour. This chapter will explore the changing fortunes of these two categories of practitioner, focusing on three main themes: the rise of the man-midwife, the use of science to overcome moral objections to the involvement of men in childbirth and the evolution of a new division of labour between the two occupational groups. Women's experience of giving birth differed in urban and rural locations, but one in seven people during this period lived in London and so the capital – where those men who practised midwifery usually trained – will feature prominently in this chapter.[5]

The Rise of the Man-Midwife

The eighteenth century was the era of the man-midwife and by mid-century it was claimed that in London 'there now are more Men-midwives than Streets'.[6] One of the most famous of these, William Smellie, declared that by 1751 his own midwifery pupils had already numbered 900,[7] and in a 1793 treatise Samuel Fores maintained that five new men-midwives had set up practice in just one street in the preceding six months.[8] Opponents argued that this expansion meant that none of these men would be able to obtain sufficient practical experience.[9] One such opponent, the midwife Elizabeth Nihell, a Catholic woman whose training included two years in France,[10] insisted that she had delivered 'above nine hundred women', making a deliberate comparison with Smellie's 900-plus students in order to demonstrate the superiority of experience in delivery over teaching others how to do it.[11]

Men-midwives – a term that came into common use from around 1720 – challenged the previously established division of labour between men, who as surgeons intervened only in difficult births, and women, who as midwives were exclusively responsible for normal births. In practice, of course, such a gendered division had always been an ideal rather than an accurate reflection of practice;

due to considerations of availability as much as money, women were often the only people present at a difficult birth. Barbara Brandon Schnorrenberg is misleading when she states that whereas the 'physician had instruments' the midwife had none;[12] midwives in the eighteenth century used not only turning of the foetus and drugs but also the crotchet or hook, the 'midwife's knife' and sometimes the fillet, a flexible noose which fitted over the head of the child, attached to a firm handle, allowing traction to be exerted. However, as we shall see, they were not normally allowed to use the forceps. In his *Observations in Midwifery*, written between 1660 and 1672, Percival Willughby explained how to use the crotchet properly, saying that bad midwives used as a substitute 'pothooks, packneedles, silver spoons, thatcher's hooks, and knives'.[13]

While women, like men, had instruments, it was the midwives' ability to prescribe drugs that was increasingly challenged in the eighteenth century. In the late seventeenth century, a mixture called 'the midwife's powder' was used to help in lengthy labours,[14] but in 1733 Edmund Chapman insisted that he would give midwives no information on medicines because that was an area exclusively for physicians.[15] In 1736 Thomas Dawkes told a trainee midwife that she should ask for advice in this area from an apothecary or 'some Man who practises Midwifery'. When she responded that 'old and experienced Midwives, all of them, have their Medicines by 'em', however, he did concede that a midwife should carry 'some good and safe Opiate' to use if needed, especially in rural areas.[16] A physician's casebook from this period noted that opiates were standard to prevent after-pains,[17] while men-midwives asserted simply, 'I gave the opiate mixture as usual', also using such drugs to suppress 'false pains'.[18]

Originally trained as surgeons, physicians or apothecaries, men-midwives claimed they could manage not just difficult births but also normal childbirth, in the place of traditional midwives. They based this claim on taking courses of instruction with established men-midwives such as Smellie. Men had in fact been involved in normal childbirth in the seventeenth century; for example, Willughby had a significant obstetric practice within a ten-mile radius of his home in Derby, and his daughter Eleanor and another family member were midwives.[19] Willughby's approach was to trust Nature, and in difficult presentations to perform podalic version or 'turning', altering the position of the foetus in the uterus so that its feet would emerge first at birth; it is likely that he learned his midwifery from the women of the family, rather than the reverse.[20] Only in the eighteenth century, however, was the term 'man-midwife' commonly applied to such men, and they needed to learn a social role as well as a new set of skills based on the anatomy of the pelvis.[21]

To its opponents, the term implied all sorts of dubious moral practices, inappropriate touching of the female body and daring but unsuccessful interventions. Nevertheless, it remained the standard label in English rather than the French *accoucheur* or neologisms, such as Edward Baynard's 'midman' or John Maubray's 'androboethogynist'.[22] Though such labels reflect how unnatural the concept of a man in this role felt to contemporaries, Lisa Forman Cody has pointed out that there was also an argument from Nature for men-midwives. The French physician Pierre Demours observed in the 1730s that the male toad appears to 'perform the function of a midwife' in assisting the female to lay her eggs; this finding appeared in English in 1753, with the conclusion that this could be seen as a natural justification for 'the practice of men-mid-wives'.[23]

As well as setting the new profession on a scientific basis, attempts were made to give it a historical pedigree.[24] Men-midwives created a lineage for themselves going back to Greco-Roman antiquity. Since there had been no men-midwives in this period, this was a difficult manoeuvre. Nevertheless, Smellie claimed that Hippocrates, the fifth-century BC 'Father of Medicine', was the Father of Midwifery.[25] Colin Mackenzie, in 1753 Smellie's senior pupil,[26] and from 1755–72 a midwifery teacher in London in his own right,[27] went so far as to call Hippocrates 'the first Man-Midwife'. He added: 'It does not appear that Hippocrates ever deliver'd any woman, and what he asserts is from theory alone, and what he acquired by being conversant with those that had Practised which was Women only, in Former ages.'[28] Other men-midwives looked to Celsus, who lived in the early Roman Empire and, like the writer of the Hippocratic treatise *On the Excision of the Foetus*, described embryotomy.[29]

Men-midwives' claims about history were reflected in the certificates given to students who completed the midwifery courses they taught in London. Up to 1743 at least, Smellie did not issue certificates, instead signing the prospectus to state that a named student had 'attend[ed] my lectures and labours'; in addition to lectures, he offered the opportunity to witness a birth. A bust of Hippocrates appeared on these certificates, while on those of other men-midwives, such as Thomas Denman in the 1770s, quotations from Celsus were used; Celsus was also cited on the title page of William Osborn's treatise on the division of the symphysis pubis.[30] This operation was a fashion of the 1770s, attacked by writers such as Freeman[31] as dangerous and unnecessary, its dire effects on women including urinary incontinence. Nihell's attack on men-midwives singled out Celsus when arguing that one should not be 'too much carried away by the authority of a great name'.[32] But he was a more appropriate hero for a man dealing only with difficult births than for the new men-midwives, and these references to him suggest that, whatever men-midwives hoped, most of their work remained on an emergency basis, concerned with difficult births.[33]

A further issue concerned the moral respectability of the man-midwife, an area focused on the key issues of touching and seeing the woman's genitalia. Ballads such as 'The Man-Midwife Unmasqu'd' (1734) played with the image of the man-midwife who warned his patient not to 'start' when he will 'search into your Treasure'.[34] 'He has rare midwife's fingers' was a proverbial (and not usually flattering) phrase,[35] but touch was considered necessary to determine pregnancy. False pains had to be distinguished from true labour; in true labour, the os would be open. Finally, touch enabled the midwife to identify the position of foetal presentation; the knee and the head were particularly easily confused.[36] Notes taken from Thomas Young's lectures in Edinburgh in 1771 show that he told his students that 'the genteeler sort of people' would be lying in bed when the man-midwife came to them, and should be touched from behind.[37] Touch was always risky. It is still unclear how far the rise of man-midwifery was due to 'genteeler' women trying to set themselves apart from the birth experiences of poor women. Writing in 1737, Sarah Stone said that 'it is become quite a Fashion' in Bristol to book men-midwives in advance of labour commencing.[38] Adrian Wilson has argued that fashion was the main driving force; Irvine Loudon instead considered that there were real improvements based on an increased understanding of the process of birth.[39] Some scholars argue for men moving into midwifery because of a lack of other economic options, while others see demand, rather than supply, as the driving force, with a shortage of women midwives, meaning that people increasingly looked elsewhere.[40]

Young told his students that any 'hasty' attempt to find the vaginal os from the rear position 'will hurt the woman, and she will entertain a bad opinion of you ... according to your doing this so is their judgement of you'. If done properly, no lubrication would be necessary.[41] Fores, attacking man-midwifery in 1793, referred to 'these sly touches' and suggested that what he called doctor-midwives changed the term 'touch' into 'trying a pain' to disguise what they were in fact doing. He expressed alarm at how many women endured 'a wanton and unnecessary exposure of the most sacred part of their persons', particularly if a man-midwife brought his pupils to witness her labour. Like Nihell, he considered that the presence of men in the birthing chamber could actually halt the process of labour.[42]

From Superstition to Science

One of the responses to concerns about morality was to emphasize that 'modern' midwifery had been founded afresh on a scientific basis; in 1777 William Moore wrote of midwifery not only as a science but as 'one of the most noble studies that ever engaged the attention of the mind'.[43] Men-midwives presented their practices as superior to those of women because they were based not on accumulated experience but on anatomical knowledge and mechanical principles, transmitted by formal training. Men-midwives commonly described women as 'ignorant of anatomy'.[44] Opponents of men-midwives argued that anatomy was irrelevant if labour was normal, so women's 'ignorance' should not stop them from dealing with normal cases; furthermore, knowledge gained from dissecting dead bodies was of little use in dealing with living ones.[45]

Men-midwives also tried to link midwifery into the tradition of anatomical illustration. Lying behind Smellie's spectacular book *A Set of Anatomical Tables*, published by subscription in 1754, was the belief that the man-midwife should be a master of anatomy. The book was intended as 22 tables 'of anatomical figures, as large as the Human Subject', many engraved by Jan van Rymsdyk. The project expanded from this original plan, eventually to 40 plates. Costs were raised by subscription.[46] Van Rymsdyk also prepared the plates for William Hunter's *The Anatomy of the Gravid Uterus* (1774). Where Smellie's atlas was very practical – 'delicacy and elegance have not been so much consulted as to have them done in a strong and distinct manner'[47] – with captions and descriptions in English, Hunter's book had text in Latin and English, and was explicitly about taste, care and beauty and the superiority of Nature to Art. Smellie moved from the normal pelvis, through early pregnancy, towards birth, but Hunter started with dissection of the uterus at full term. In Hunter, the foetus is intact, with hair shown in detail, but the women's bodies are like slabs of meat – dead, but not decomposed.[48] The child is treated tenderly: the mother is mutilated. In a famous analogy, Hunter compared the anatomist with the general, knowing the features of the landscape – the 'lakes, rivers, marshes, mountains, precipices, plains, woods, roads, passes, fords, towns, fortifications etc.'. In a 1779 pamphlet, Francis Foster condemned man-midwifery because it placed the 'citadel' of female virtue 'directly in the hands of the enemy' and left it 'entirely at his discretion'.[49] The bodies in Hunter's atlas have clearly been defeated.

A further way of making midwifery scientific was to change the way it was taught. This involved creating a stereotype of the 'ignorant midwife' of the past, and arguing that women were untrained, or untrainable. Historians have long since put such stereotypes to rest.[50] We know that seventeenth-century midwives were supposed to read two books under the guidance of a senior midwife; an unpublished manuscript from the 1660s or 1670s, Edward Poeton's *The Midwives Deputie*,[51] names these as Jacques Guillemeau and the *Birth of Mankind*, while in 1736 Dawkes described a midwife whose senior midwife recommended 'Chamberlain's Midwifery' and 'Daventer'.[52] Doreen Evenden's detailed archival research shows that midwives in seventeenth-century London could spend seven years attending deliveries with a senior midwife before taking primary responsibility for them. The licensing of English midwives switched between the church and the state in this period, although practices differed between London and the provinces.[53]

A shift from focusing on the character of the midwife – often vouched for by women in her community – to looking at her knowledge seems to have begun in the late seventeenth century. Elizabeth Francis was licensed in 1690 to practise both surgery and midwifery in London, and testimonials came not from satisfied clients or her fellow midwives, but from two physicians, a surgeon and a surgeon/man-midwife.[54] At the end of the eighteenth century, some opponents of men–midwives insisted that, although there were certainly some bad midwives in rural areas, those in London and other major cities were often very skilled, although less so under the training of men than they were when they were trained by other women.[55] Stone, who published a book of her midwifery cases in 1737, was trained by her mother, Mrs Holmes, and acted as deputy to her for six years, rating what she learned from her above the knowledge gained from reading or from witnessing dissections.[56]

Men in England could receive some training in midwifery as part of a medical degree, although it was not compulsory. In the eighteenth century, however, they also took specialized training courses open to all who were willing to pay, not only to surgeons, apothecaries and physicians, but also – in some cases – to women. From this mixing of previously separate disciplines, it has been argued that the general practitioner would eventually emerge.[57] Would-be men-midwives sometimes attended the lectures given by more than one expert in the field, and took repeat courses. Robert Wallace Johnson, for example, referred to having attended Smellie's lectures in 1750,[58] and the diary of Richard Kay, a Lancashire surgeon who returned to a rural practice, shows that he took two courses with Smellie in 1744, at the end of a year of training in London at Guy's Hospital.[59]

This pattern of taking a midwifery course only at the end of one's London training was later condemned by John Leake, who wrote in 1773 that it was better to take it earlier, alongside the anatomy training.[60] Some men, such as Denman, ran private courses as well as holding a post at a teaching hospital.[61] Those offering courses advertised on 'gilt boards' outside their homes.[62] Smellie himself took advantage of the new medium of the day, the newspaper, to advertise his courses and books more widely. After 1720, the number of advertisements in newspapers grew significantly as the number of titles increased; by the 1780s there were at least nine daily newspapers, eight tri-weekly and approximately nine weekly papers in London, with the tri-weekly ones also being sent to the provinces.[63] This significantly increased the audience for man-midwifery.

Smellie, who taught in London between 1739 and 1758, was one of the most famous men-midwives of this period. A surgeon-apothecary, from 1724 or earlier, he was called in by local midwives and families to help at the final stages of difficult births, concentrating exclusively on midwifery from 1737. His most important contribution to understanding the mechanical basis of midwifery was his understanding of how the foetal head turns in the birth canal. He taught this using what he called 'machines': real skeletons of the female pelvis, with ligaments, muscles and skin made of artificial materials, together with cloth dolls. Different machines were used for different problems, such as the 'Circumstances of the Child', 'the Narrowness of the Bones of the Mother' and so on.[64] One doll had a head that separated from the body to demonstrate how to manage if the head remained in the uterus after the rest of the body had been extracted with instruments.

The syllabus of Smellie's course in 1742 shows that the 'Machines' were in regular use, alongside 'wet and dry Preparations, and other artificial Contrivances';[65] he also developed artificial wombs with hinges, some also having glass windows.[66] Smellie was by no means the only man-midwife using machines: Sir Richard Manningham used a 'great machine' as well as a 'glass machine'.[67] In around 1770, Denman and Osborn jointly purchased for £120 the 'apparatus' of a teacher of midwifery called Dr Cooper.[68] Similar models were used in displays open to the paying public in London from the 1730s; for example, a wax womb 'laid open at the Top, and therein you see the little inhabitant endeavouring to quit his Prison, and be released' – a reference to the ancient belief that labour is initiated by the child's attempts to escape from the womb, the labouring woman being passive.[69]

Accounts survive from contemporaries who saw Smellie's machines in use, and his students and successors praised them because they meant that 'every material circumstance might be laid open to the naked Eye'.[70] But opponents found them unconvincing. Nihell famously dismissed them as 'a mere wooden machine' or 'a wooden statue', in which 'a bladder full, perhaps, of small beer, represented the uterus', with the baby as 'a wax-doll' or 'an artificial doll'.[71] William Douglas noted that they were made of 'natural Bones', but with 'the Addition of Shoes, Stockings, and the common Apparel of Women, but of what Use are these to the Learner?'[72] However, other opponents of men-midwifery considered the machines a far better way of teaching men-midwives than learning on living women.[73]

Knowledge of the birth process was complemented by the use of the forceps, to mimic the natural turning of the child in the birth canal. Originally kept as a secret within the Chamberlen family, they were introduced to a wider public by Chapman's 1733 treatise.[74] When the first male forceps-users sold the secret to the next generation, they did not always explain precisely how to use this instrument, and so there were a series of disastrous failures; for example, the forceps would 'slip' and come out.[75] History was invoked in defence of forceps use. 'Ancient' and 'modern' in this period were normally aligned with women's midwifery as 'ancient', men's practice (with instruments) as 'modern'. In the case of forceps, the aim was rather different: to show that male intervention in normal delivery was in fact 'ancient'.

Some eighteenth-century men-midwives such as Osborn and Denman told their students that 'the forceps is a very old instrument', while others such as Young told his that 'This is a modern instrument, invented about a century ago.'[76] The key point was what was meant by forceps: the extraction forceps was indeed old, but the forceps used to deliver a living child, without loss of the mother, was a new device. Women entered these debates: Nihell, an outspoken enemy of the man-midwife, also regarded the forceps as new, saying that the midwives of her time were 'indebted to the moderns for it'.[77]

Some eighteenth-century men-midwives such as Brudenell Exton argued that what the Chamberlens had kept as their family secret was not the forceps, but 'a manual operation' – that of turning the baby to the feet-first position; this continued to be recommended as the best action to take in anything other than a head-first presentation.[78] The eighteenth-century man-midwife was not necessarily an enthusiastic user of the forceps. Johnson learned their use from Smellie, but quickly abandoned the instrument in his own practice.[79] Smellie himself changed his opinions about the forceps over the course of his career, sometimes deserting the instrument altogether, sometimes adjusting the design as a result of the difficulties he encountered. He believed that, in normal labour, 'in most cases we shall have nothing else to do but receive the child',[80] advising never to use the forceps except when absolutely necessary.[81] In 1745 Smellie had a breakthrough, finding a way of moving the forceps from side to side in a head-first delivery. He expressed his 'great joy' that 'my eyes were now opened to a new field of improvement, on the method of using the forceps in this position'.[82]

While the forceps, if properly used, meant that the presence of a man in the birthing-chamber was no longer necessarily a signal that a death would take place, women in labour still took some convincing. As the English translation of Dionis (1719) has it, 'The very sight of 'em fills not only the mother, but all who are present with horror.'[83] At one period of Smellie's life, he even experimented with leather-covered forceps in order not to alarm women with the metallic clank of the blades.

Men-midwives were not a cohesive group; their published case histories reveal a complex picture of inter-professional rivalry and cooperation, with each other and with other groups. Wilson has shown how those favouring forceps tended to be Tories and hence associated with 'traditional' values, while those who avoided intervention were Whigs and hence associated with 'progressive' values. Sometimes men allied themselves on party lines, but often they simply tried to stay off each other's turf. In 1742 Smellie reported that he was called to a woman who 'had been four times delivered by another gentleman of dead children'. He commented that 'I was averse to interfere with any other practitioner' but, when assured that this gentleman would not be employed again, took the case, although he did advise the patient to consult a physician for her 'icterical complaints', or jaundice.[84]

Wilson has demonstrated that, under the umbrella of 'man-midwifery', several different modes of intervention existed. He distinguished between advance, onset and emergency calls.[85] In advance calls, the midwife would stay in the house until the birth began, so that only the very rich could consider an advance call. There was also the distinction between being booked (or 'bespoke') and unbooked. Smellie was 'several times bespoke to attend women in their first children, by their friends, who were apprehensive, that they would have difficult or dangerous labours, because they were distorted in their backs'.[86] He could take a few hours of sleep at the house he was visiting, leaving a nurse or midwife with the woman under strict instructions to call him if her condition changed.

Those booked by the gentry or the middling sort could be hired even for emergency calls, and on attending the birth may – or may not – find that a midwife had also been employed. One of Smellie's pupils was bespoke to a woman who also employed a midwife, keeping him in reserve 'in case any extraordinary incident should intervene', and when things did not proceed well Smellie was summoned by his pupil.[87] However, as Smellie could not attend immediately, the midwife called in another man-midwife. He recommended delivery by the fillet, while Smellie successfully urged that the forceps should be used. While only the well-off could afford a booked call, unbooked emergency calls could be to women from any economic background, and often came free of charge.[88]

Midwives and Men-Midwives

Because many men-midwives were called only for emergency cases, it was important that they were known and trusted by the midwives who would decide when a woman could not be delivered naturally. Smellie noted that 'When midwifery came to be more practised by gentlemen than formerly, one Dr C__, visited all the midwives, and left printed notes of his abode.'[89] When Smellie praised midwives, it was usually for their acute powers of observation or for their sense in calling him in. He needed somebody to tell him clearly what had happened before his arrival. In one of his cases, 'the people about her' claimed a woman had been in labour eight days; 'they said, three midwives had attended and left her'.[90] His ideal midwife was 'a decent, sensible woman of a middle age' who understood the structure of the pelvis and knew how to detect foetal position by touch; in other words, one who shared the knowledge on which men-midwives based their practice.[91] He had 'his' midwives, some known to have been taught by him, who waited with women who had booked him until it was time to call Smellie himself at the start of the final stage of labour; his midwives remained with him as he performed his interventions. He referred to Mrs Maddocks (later Mrs Ward)[92] as 'my midwife', and used her to monitor laborious cases when he had to be elsewhere, or even to deliver 'on my account'.[93] Writing in 1764, Philip Thicknesse also praised the work of 'Mrs Draper, Mrs Maddox, and many other women' who could do all that was needed in delivery.[94] Smellie mentions Mrs Draper by name, but does not say that he taught her.[95]

It is clear that the ideal midwife knew her limitations.[96] In 1751, Exton wrote to teach women midwives 'what is their proper Business, and what not', while all were agreed that, in the words of Chapman, writing in 1753, 'The best Midwives commonly send for Advice upon the Appearance of Danger.'[97] But by cultivating his relationships with midwives, never 'openly condemning her method of practice, (even though it should be erroneous)',[98] Smellie could be the man-midwife of choice in difficult cases. He observed that 'Another gentleman, many years ago, made a great bustle, got into a considerable share of practice by taking low prices. He abused the midwives, right or wrong, and was abused by them.'[99] Because of his scare tactics, he 'frightened man midwives from calling in menpractitioners'.[100] An anonymous man-midwife contemporary with Smellie criticized a midwife who tried to speed up the delivery so that it would be completed before he arrived, describing the death of both mother and child as 'the consequences of the folly, rashness and selfishness of an impudent woman'.[101] Experience, praised by many opponents of the man-midwife as the 'best Instructor',[102] was not seen as any guarantee of competence; a midwife of 36 years experience whom he encountered in 1742 was still 'a very ignorant woman' and 'a Brute'.[103]

But it would be wrong to emphasize the alleged failings of midwives. Men-midwives were just as likely to be criticized, and even brought to court. In a famous case of 1754 tried at the Guildhall in London, Richard Maddox sued for £5000 damages against Dr Matthew Morley, a physician and man-midwife, for refusing to come to help his wife in May 1753; the child was dead and Mrs Maddox died three months later. A midwife, Mrs Hopkins, described in the trial as 'a woman of great experience and reputation' 'honestly told' Maddox that she could not help, and so Morley was sent for, having successfully delivered Mrs Maddox four years previously. The family's apothecary, Dr Langley, was also present. Morley agreed Mrs Maddox was in a serious condition, and announced that he was going home, promising to return later. But when called out later that day, he refused to return. Another doctor, Dr Hannakin, was called but refused to proceed until he had support, so Dr Middleton was also called. The case hinged on Morley's claim that he was attending as a physician – not as a man-midwife – and that this was why he had not stayed; when called the second time he said he had not been fit to come out. Another man-midwife, Dr Sands, gave him a good character reference, but argued that he should have attended. The jury found against Morley but restricted the damages to £1000.[104] Smellie himself was involved in a very similar case a few years previously, in which Morley had been bespoke, but refused to come out because he was with another case.[105]

We can see more of the political dimensions of the birthing chamber in a case of 1748. Douglas claimed that he was the first on the scene, called for by the woman's husband, and that he had sent for Dr Wilmot to assist him. In the interim, however, somebody else had already called Smellie.[106] Smellie did not accept Douglas's prognosis, and called as witness 'Mr Bromfield, Apothecary'.[107] A fourth player then entered this crowded birth chamber: a physician, Dr Wilmot.[108] Drugs had been given to the woman by Bromfield, and the disagreement between Smellie and Douglas hinged on whether a lethargic woman should be left in the hope that normal contractions would resume, or whether intervention with the forceps should be tried immediately, although it would not necessarily save the child.

At least for some women, the rise of the lying-in hospital, beginning with the Lying-in Hospital for Married Women, opened in 1749 in London, but soon spread to the provinces, moved birth outside the home.[109] Evenden has argued that this institutional provision was 'the single most important factor in the demise of the authority and superiority of the female midwife'.[110] However, midwives continued to manage most births, even if under the supervision of men; and home births continued even in London, where the Royal Maternity Charity (RMC) was set up in 1757 to supply midwives for home deliveries, and some parishes employed their own midwife.[111] The stated purpose of hospitals such as Manningham's short-lived General Lying-in Hospital (founded next to his home in Jermyn Street, London, in 1739), or the lying-in ward at the Middlesex Hospital opened in 1747, was to provide poor women with somewhere to give birth, and then to regain their strength. But these hospitals also gave men access to women's bodies, on which they could practise their skills, as normal births there were handled by midwives, difficult births by the physician.[112]

In his attack on man-midwifery as unnecessary, Fores argued that rich women were less likely to have difficulty giving birth, so that men-midwives, even if necessary for poor women in lying-in hospitals, should not be needed by the rich.[113] More commonly, rich women were seen as so far from the natural state of woman that they were likely to have problems in giving birth.[114] Ethnicity also featured in this discourse. The slave trade meant that British doctors were examining the bodies of Africans, which led to comparisons between the two races and to medical concern about the progeny of mixed-race marriages; could they themselves reproduce? Though opposing the slave trade, Charles White, a surgeon and man-midwife who helped set up the Manchester Lying-in Hospital in 1790, argued for the superiority of 'whites' over 'blacks' in intellectual and aesthetic terms.[115] It was noticed – or at least alleged – that non-European women gave birth more easily; for example, John Coakley Lettsom claimed that women in a 'southern climate' usually had no pain in childbirth.[116] This ease of giving birth was linked to people of non-European races having not only larger pelvises, but also smaller heads.[117]

Was the new scientific midwifery that articulated these ideas available to women pupils? Women were trained by the great London men-midwifery instructors, but in separate classes. Fores suggested that men-midwives charged women 12 guineas without teaching them how to turn, and accepted fees from those who could not possibly benefit from the instruction.[118] In 1751, Smellie considered that a woman could 'hardly be supposed mistress of all these qualifications' that a man could attain, but she should be 'perfectly well instructed with regard to the bones of the pelvis . . . well skilled in the method of touching pregnant women . . . perfectly mistress in the art of examination in time of labour'.[119] At the end of this period, Smellie's principles were being taught to women, by women. Margaret Stephen, 'Teacher of Midwifery to Females', who after 30 years in practice published a midwifery book in 1795, stated that she was 'taught by a gentleman, who had been a pupil of Dr Smellie'. She learned 'the principles upon which nature acted, and the mechanical powers, by which she must be assisted, when deficient'. Midwifery, she insisted, was a 'science',[120] but it was one that could be taught to women.

Stephen regarded her own pupils as being 'as well qualified as men', taught by her 'the anatomy of the pelvis, &c' 'on preparations which I keep by me', how to turn a baby and even how to use the forceps and other instruments. On forceps, she commented, 'there is none of all the instruments I ever saw, so well calculated to save the lives of children'. She told her female pupils exactly how to insert the instrument to grip the head properly, but recommended that they call in someone else if it were necessary to use the forceps, simply to transfer the blame 'should any misfortune happen'. While in difficult cases she was in favour of calling in a physician to assist the midwife, she did not support men-midwives, suggesting that most of these were originally apothecaries only. In one case she described, a slow labour so alarmed the labouring woman's friends and family that they insisted on calling in someone else. This practitioner, a young and inexperienced apothecary with 'man-midwife' on his door, was described scathingly as 'a perfect twig of the obstetric profession'. A wound on the temple of the dead baby which he delivered with his forceps suggested to Stephen that the process of delivery killed it.[121]

Conclusion

Despite Stephen's best efforts, at the end of the eighteenth century the midwife's position had deteriorated significantly. There were several reasons. Moral objections to men-midwives had been overcome; their use had become a badge of gentility for at least some families from the upper and middling classes; and the scientific foundations for practice, pivotal to professionalization, were being developed. The arrival of the lying-in hospital as an institutional locus for care compounded the influence of these trends. But although the basic principle that men could and even should manage normal birth had been established, the division of labour within midwifery was far from rigidly gendered. Women had access to the new scientific knowledge through training, albeit increasingly provided by female midwives. More significantly, they functioned within an inter-professional relationship that was critical to the men-midwives, who relied on women's specialist expertise to identify emergencies.

Notes

1. L. Forman Cody, *Birthing the Nation: Sex, Science, and the Conception of Eighteenth-Century Britons* (Oxford: Oxford University Press, 2005).

On the provinces, see D. Harley, 'Provincial Midwives in England: Lancashire and Cheshire, 1660–1760', in H. Marland (ed.), *The Art of Midwifery: Early Modern Midwives in Europe* (London: Routledge, 1993) pp. 27–48; S. S. Thomas, 'Early Modern Midwifery: Splitting the Profession, Connecting the History', *Journal of Social History*, 43 (2009) 115–38.

2. J.C. Lettsom, *History of the Origin of Medicine: An Oration to the Medical Society of London, January 19, 1778* (London: J. Phillips, 1778) note to p. 48; W. Smellie, *A Collection of Cases and Observations in Midwifery* (London: D. Wilson and T. Durham, 1754) pp. 235, 238–9.

3. A. Shepard, 'The Literature of a Medical Hoax: The Case of Mary Toft, the Pretended Rabbet-Breeder', *Eighteenth-Century Life*, 19 (1995) 59–77; L. Forman Cody, 'The Doctor's in Labour; or a New Whim-Wham from Guildford', *Gender and History*, 4 (1992) 175–96.

4. P. Dionis, *A General Treatise of Midwifery* (London: A. Bell et al., 1719) pp. 254–5.

5. Cody, *Birthing the Nation*, p. ix.

6. W. Douglas, *A Letter to Dr Smelle [sic] Shewing the Impropriety of His New-invented Wooden Forceps: As Also, the Absurdity of His Method of Teaching and Practising Midwifery* (London: J. Roberts, 1748) pp. 5–6.

7. Smellie, *Cases and Observations*, p. v.

8. Samuel Fores writing as 'John Blunt', *Man-Midwifery Dissected; or, the Obstetric Family-Instructor. For the Use of Married Couples, and Single Adults of Both Sexes* (London: Samuel William Fores, 1793) p. 49.

9. Douglas, *A Letter to Dr Smelle*, pp. 5–6.

10. Cody, *Birthing the Nation*, pp. 184–5.

11. E. Nihell, *A Treatise on the Art of Midwifery* (London: A. Morley, 1760) p. 50.

12. B. Brandon Schnorrenberg, 'Is Childbirth any Place for a Woman? The Decline of Midwifery in Eighteenth-century England', *Studies in Eighteenth-Century Culture*, 10 (1981) 393–408, reprinted in E. R. Van Teijlingen, G. W. Lowis, P. McCaffery and M. Porter (eds), *Midwifery and the Medicalization of Childbirth: Comparative Perspectives* (New York: Nova Science Publishers, 2004) p. 90.

13. P. Willughby, *Observations in Midwifery* (Wakefield: C.R. Publishers, reprint of 1863 edition, Warwick: H.T. Cooke, 1972) p. 151.

14. Willughby, *Observations*, p. 82; recipe p. 60.

15. E. Chapman, *An Essay towards the Improvement of Midwifery* (London: A. Blackwell, 1733) Preface.

16. T. Dawkes, *The Midwife Rightly Instructed* (London: J. Oswald, 1736), p. 9; reprinted in Stephen Freeman, *The Ladies Friend* (London: printed for the author, 1787), pp. 291 ff., pp. 37–41.

17. Royal College of Physicians of Edinburgh [RCPEd.], Manuscript [Ms.] Anon. 24: Casebook 1739–50, 'Cases and Observations in Midwifery by a Practitioner in Surrey', p. 100, case 88.

18. B. Exton, *A New and General System of Midwifery in Four Parts* (London: W. Owen, 1751) p. 46.

19. A. Wilson, 'A Memorial of Eleanor Willughby, a Seventeenth-Century Midwife', in L. Hunter and S. Hutton (eds), *Women, Science and Medicine 1500–1700: Mothers and Sisters of the Royal Society* (Stroud: Sutton, 1997) pp. 138–77.

20. D. Evenden, *The Midwives of Seventeenth-Century London* (Cambridge and New York: Cambridge University Press, 2000) p. 182.

21. A. Wilson, 'William Hunter and the Varieties of Man-Midwifery', in W. F. Bynum and R. Porter (eds), *William Hunter and the Eighteenth-Century Medical World* (Cambridge: Cambridge University Press, 1985) p. 362; G. B. Risse, *New Medical Challenges during the Scottish Enlightenment* (Amsterdam: Rodopi, 2005) p. 286.

22. A. Wilson, *The Making of Man-Midwifery: Childbirth in England, 1660–1770* (Cambridge: Harvard University Press, 1995) pp. 107–8.

23. P. Templeman (ed.), *Curious Remarks and Observations . . . Extracted from the History and Memoirs of the Royal Academy of Sciences at Paris*, 2 vols (1753), i.371–4 cited in Cody, *Birthing the Nation*, p. 247.

24. Wilson, 'William Hunter'.

25. W. Smellie, *A Treatise on the Theory and Practice of Midwifery*, 2nd edition, corrected (London: D. Wilson, 1752) p. iv; Lucinda Macray Beier, *Sufferers and Healers: The Experience of Illness in Seventeenth-Century England* (London and New York: Routledge and Kegan Paul, 1988) p. 44; H. King, *Midwifery, Obstetrics and the Rise of Gynaecology. The Uses of a Sixteenth-Century Compendium* (Aldershot and Burlington, VT: Ashgate, 2007) p. 99.

26. Mackenzie is described as 'senior pupil' in W. Smellie, *A Collection of Preternatural Cases and Observations in Midwifery* (London: D. Wilson and T. Durham, 1764) p. 305.

27. Lecture notes from his classes survive. Wellcome Library, Ms. Wellc. 3392, 'Dr MacKenzie's Lectures' and Ms. Wellc. MSL 110, 'Ars Obstetricandi', a further, undated, set of notes from MacKenzie's lectures formerly incorrectly attributed in the catalogue to Thomas Young. The dates for his teaching are taken from S. C. Lawrence, *Charitable Knowledge: Hospital Pupils and Practitioners in Eighteenth-Century London* (Cambridge: Cambridge University Press, 1996) Appendix 3.

28. Ms. Wellc. 3392, pp. 65, 6, 1–2, dated to 1770 on internal evidence. See also Ms. Wellc. MSL 110, pp. 1, 5.

29. Celsus, *De medicina*, 7.29.

30. W. Osborn, *An Essay on Laborious Parturition: In Which the Division of the Symphysis Pubis Is Particularly Considered* (London: T. Cadell, 1783).

31. Freeman, *Ladies Friend*, pp. 117–18.

32. Nihell, *Art of Midwifery*, p. 369.

33. Wilson, 'William Hunter', p.357.

34. 'The Man-Midwife Unmasqu'd' (London: J. Dormer, 1734).
35. Nihell, *Art of Midwifery*, p. 111.
36. Exton, *New and General System*, pp. 44, 80.
37. Royal College of Surgeons of England [RCSEng.], Ms. Young, Notes, vol. 1, p. 4.
38. S. Stone, *A Complete Practice of Midwifery. Consisting of Upwards of Forty Cases or Observations in that Valuable Art . . .* (London: Printed for T. Cooper, 1737), p. x; I. Grundy, 'Sarah Stone: Enlightenment Midwife', in R. Porter (ed.), *Medicine in the Enlightenment* (Amsterdam: Rodopi, 1995).
39. Wilson, *Making of Man-Midwifery*; I. S. L. Loudon, 'Essay Review: The Making of Man-Midwifery', *Bulletin of the History of Medicine*, 70 (1996) 507–15.
40. A. Wilson, 'Midwifery in the "medical marketplace"', in M. Jenner and P. Wallis (eds), *Medicine and the Market in England and Its Colonies, c. 1450–c. 1850* (Basingstoke: Palgrave Macmillan, 2007) p. 158.
41. RCSEng., Ms. Young, Notes, p. 7.
42. Fores, *Man-Midwifery Dissected*, pp. xvi, 31–3, 48; Nihell, *Art of Midwifery*, pp. 235–6.
43. W. Moore, *Elements of Midwifery, or the Arcana of Nature* (London: J. Johnson, 1777), p. 226.
44. E.g. Thomas Young lectures 1774, Ms. Wellc. 5108, p. 3.
45. Stone, *Complete Practice of Midwifery*, pp. xi–xii; Fores, *Man-Midwifery Dissected*, p. 165.
46. *London Evening Post*, Tuesday, 25 February 1752.
47. W. Smellie, *A Set of Anatomical Tables, with Explanations, and an Abridgment, of the Practice of Midwifery, with a View to Illustrate a Treatise on that Subject, and Collection of Cases* (London: [D. Wilson] 1754), p. iv.
48. L. Jordanova, 'Gender, Generation and Science: William Hunter's Anatomical Atlas', in W. F. Bynum and R. Porter (eds), *William Hunter and the Eighteenth-Century Medical World* (Illinois: University of Chicago Press, 1985) p. 388.
49. F. Foster, *Thoughts on the Times: But Chiefly on the Profligacy of our Women, and it's Causes* (London, 1779), pp. 79–80 and 196–7; L. Massey, 'Dissecting Pregnancy in Eighteenth-Century Europe', http://anatomyofgender.northwestern.edu/massey01.html#foot, accessed 16 November 2009.
50. D. Harley, 'Ignorant Midwives – A Persistent Stereotype', *Bulletin of the Society for the Social History of Medicine*, 28 (1981) 6–9.
51. British Library [BL], Ms., Sloane 1954, 9v.
52. Dawkes, *Midwife Rightly Instructed*, p. 9; reprinted in Freeman, *Ladies Friend*, pp. 291 with the midwife Lucina renamed Sophia.
53. Wilson, 'Midwifery in the "medical marketplace"', pp. 156, 164.

54. Evenden, *Midwives*, pp. 176–7.
55. Fores, *Man-Midwifery Dissected*, pp. 174–5; 178.
56. Stone, *Complete Practice of Midwifery*, pp. xv and xxiii. Grundy, 'Sarah Stone', p. 129.
57. I. S. L. Loudon, *Medical Care and the General Practitioner, 1750–1850* (Oxford: Clarendon Press, 1986) p. 90; Evenden, *Midwives*, p. 176.
58. R.W Johnson, *A New System of Midwifery, in Four Parts; Founded on Practical Observations: The Whole Illustrated with Copper Plates* (London: printed for the author, 1769) pp. 172–3.
59. See W. Brockbank and M. L. Kay, 'Extracts from the Diary of Richard Kay of Baldington, Bury, Surgeon', *Medical History*, 3 (1959) 58–68; W. Brockbank and F. Kenworthy, *The Diary of Richard Kay, 1716–51: Of Baldingstone, Near Bury, a Lancashire Doctor* (Manchester: Manchester University Press, 1968).
60. J. Leake, *A Syllabus of Lectures on the Theory and Practice of Midwifery* (London, 1776) p. 2.
61. Ms. Wellc. 5620, 'Life of Dr Denman', p. 8.
62. Freeman, *Ladies Friend*, p. 90.
63. H. Barker, *Newspapers, Politics and Public Opinion in Late Eighteenth-Century England* (Oxford: Clarendon Press, 1998) p. 23.
64. Smellie, *Collection of Cases*, p. 354; Anon., *A Catalogue of the Entire and Inestimable Apparatus for Lectures in Midwifery, Contrived with Consummate Judgment, and Executed with Infinite Labour, by the Late Ingenious Dr William Smellie, Deceased* (London: no publisher stated, 1770) p. 6.
65. Ms. Wellc. 4630. Some of the 'wet and dry preparations' were also sold in 1770. See *A Catalogue of the Entire and Inestimable Apparatus for Lectures in Midwifry*, pp. 4–5.
66. *A Catalogue of the Entire and Inestimable Apparatus for Lectures in Midwifry*, p. 6.
67. R. Manningham, *An Abstract of Midwifery, for the Use of the Lying-in Infirmary* (London: T. Gardner, 1744) p.15.
68. Ms. Wellc. 5620, 'Life of Dr Denman', p. 7.
69. *A Catalogue and Particular Description of the Human Anatomy in Wax-Work, and Several Other Preparations to Be Seen at the Royal-Exchange* (London, 1736), p. 13. On the widespread belief in the 'increased strugglings, or motion of the child' as the cause of labour see, for example, Freeman, *The Ladies Friend* (4th edition, 1785) p. 173.
70. Manuscript, Royal College of Physicians of England [Ms. RCPEd.] 'Notes on Midwifery', classified as Young, T. 8, pp. 2–3. Colin Mackenzie praised the machines, and also continued to use them (Wellc. Ms. 3392, pp. 6, 122).
71. Nihell, *Art of Midwifery*, pp. 50, 51, 71.
72. W. Douglas, *A Second Letter to Dr. Smelle* [*sic*]*, and an Answer to his Pupil, Confirming the Impropriety of His Wooden Forceps; As Also of His*

Method of Teaching and Practising Midwifery (London: S. Paterson, 1748) pp. 24–5; J. Glaister, *Smellie and His Contemporaries: A Contribution to the History of Midwifery in the Eighteenth Century* (Glasgow: Maclehose, 1894) pp. 89–97.

73. Fores, *Man-Midwifery Dissected*, p. 81.
74. Chapman, *Essay towards the Improvement of Midwifery*.
75. Smellie, *Collection of Cases* 1764, p. 326. The third edition. London, 1764.
76. King's College London, Ms. KCL TH/PP5, p. 110; RCSEng., Ms.Young, p. 60.
77. Nihell, *Art of Midwifery*, p. 42.
78. Exton, *New and General System*, p. 5.
79. Johnson, *A New System of Midwifery*, pp. 172–3.
80. Smellie, *Collection of Cases*, pp. 233, 228–44, are devoted to natural labours, although in many cases described here, the child is nevertheless stillborn.
81. Smellie, *Collection of Cases* (1764) p. 259.
82. Smellie, *Collection of Cases* (1764) pp. 473–5.
83. Dionis, *General Treatise of Midwifery*, p. 247.
84. Smellie, *Collection of Cases* (1764) p. 366.
85. Wilson, 'William Hunter', p. 349.
86. Smellie, *Collection of Cases* (1764) p. 8.
87. Smellie, *Collection of Cases* (1764) pp. 506–7.
88. Loudon, *Medical Care*, p. 96.
89. Smellie, *Preternatural Cases*, p. 378.
90. Smellie, *Collection of Cases* (1764), p. 337.
91. Smellie, *Theory and Practice of Midwifery*, p. 448.
92. Glaister, *Smellie and his Contemporaries*, p. 48.
93. Smellie, *Collection of Cases* (1764), p.365. William Smellie, *Preternatural Cases*, p. 382. On Mrs Maddocks/Maddox, see Glaister, *Smellie and His Contemporaries*, p. 48. In eighteenth-century midwifery language, 'Laborious' is usually the term for labour lasting for more than 24 hours.
94. Thicknesse, *Man-Midwifery Analysed*, p. 25.
95. Smellie, *Theory and Practice of Midwifery*, p. 447, Case 3.
96. Manningham, *An Abstract of Midwifery*, p. 16.
97. Exton, *New and General System*, p. 11; Chapman, *A Treatise on the Improvement of Midwifery* (3rd edition), p. xviii.
98. Smellie, *Theory and Practice of Midwifery*, pp. 448–9.
99. Smellie, *Preternatural Cases*, p. 378.
100. Smellie, *Preternatural Cases*, p. 379.
101. RCPEd., Ms., Anon. 24, p.6 Case 4.
102. Foster, *Thoughts on the times*, p. 96.
103. RCPEd., Ms., Anon. 24, p. 1 Case 1.

104. R. Maddox, *The Trial of a Cause between Richard Maddox, Gent. Plaintiff, and Dr. M—y, Defendant, Physician and Man-Midwife, before Sir Michael Foster, ... At Guildhall, London, March 2, 1754....* (London, 1754), pp. 7, 9.

105. *Preternatural Cases*, pp. 142–7. Glaister identifies the anonymous practitioner here as Morley.

106. Douglas, *Second Letter to Dr. Smelle*, pp. 7–10. Also Smellie, *Preternatural Cases*, pp. 537–8.

107. *An Answer to a Late Pamphlet*, pp. 11–12. His presence is also noted in Douglas, *Second Letter to Dr. Smelle*, p. 10.

108. In this high-profile case, this was probably Edward Wilmot, who was physician to the household of Prince Frederick from 1742 to 1751; the role had been held by Francis Clifton from 1730 to 1734. See the list of the Prince's household at http://www.history.ac.uk/office/fred_alpha.html accessed 14 November 2005.

109. For a useful diagram showing the development of the London lying-in hospitals, see Wilson, *Making of Man-Midwifery*, p. 146, figure 11.1.

110. Evenden, *Midwives*, p. 180.

111. Cody, *Birthing the Nation,* pp. 176–7, 184.

112. Manningham, *An Abstract of Midwifery*, p. 34; Wilson, *Making of Man-Midwifery*, p. 145.

113. Fores, *Man-Midwifery Dissected*, pp. 48–9.

114. E.g. T. Denman, *An Introduction to the Practice of Midwifery* Vol. 2 (London: T. Bensley for J. Johnson, 1788) p. 117.

115. Cody, *Birthing the Nation*, pp. 238–9.

116. J.C. Lettsom, 'History of the Origin of Medicine: An Oration', *Medical Society of London*, January 19, 1778.

117. C. White, *An Account of the Regular Gradation in Man* (London: C. Dilly, 1799), cited in Cody, *Birthing the Nation*, pp. 251–2.

118. Fores, *Man-Midwifery Dissected*, pp. 51, 179–80.

119. Smellie, *Theory and Practice of Midwifery*, Book IV, Chapter 3, Section 2, 'Of the Midwife'.

120. Stephen, *Domestic Midwife*, pp. 17–19.

121. Stephen, *Domestic Midwife*, pp. 4, 43, 58, 69–70, 86.

6

Midwifery, 1800–1920: The Journey to Registration

Alison Nuttall

In 1843, midwife Christian Cowper died a fortnight after her last case, the 3,948[th] in the book in which she recorded every delivery she attended in a well-educated hand. Trained in Edinburgh by Alexander Hamilton, then the only British professor of midwifery, she had built up a successful practice over 57 years in Thurso, despite the presence of three doctors: indeed, she counted their wives among her clients.[1] Four years later, Mary Eaves, a weaver's wife, began her practice in Coventry. A mother of seven, it is unclear how she learned her midwifery. Although equally successful, delivering 4,438 babies in 35 years, Mrs Eaves embodied the perceived deterioration in the nineteenth-century midwife: her clients were her neighbours in a poor area; she was illiterate, unable to sign the marriage register, and reliant on assistance to complete her casebook.[2] Five years after Mrs Eaves died, in 1881, Mary Ann Eleanor Stephens took the written and oral examinations for the Diploma of the Obstetrical Society of London, having previously trained at the City of London Lying-In Hospital. She went on to become 'an exceedingly successful midwife, popular ... with patients and doctors', who, in 28 years of practice, delivered over 8,000 infants. Although Mrs Stephens had much in common with her predecessors, as a senior member of the Midwives' Institute she also became 'Number 1' on the Midwives Roll of the Central Midwives' Board, 'entitled by law to practise as a Midwife in accordance with the provisions of the Midwives Act 1902'.[3] She died in 1910, the year that entry to the profession became by examination only. Just as the careers of these three midwives span the nineteenth century, so their experiences reflect the changes that the profession as a whole underwent in this period.

Initial examinations of the nineteenth-century development of professional midwifery focused on the work of the Midwives' Institute in achieving the successful passage through parliament of the Midwives' Act, thereby providing the profession with both origin myth and heroines, notably Zepherina Veitch and Rosalind Paget.[4] The Institute's claim to be acting in the best interests of mothers, and its assumption that it represented all right-thinking midwives, was accepted unquestioningly, and material was drawn largely from the Reports of the 1892 and 1893 Select Committees on Midwife Registration, Institute archives and its journal *Nursing Notes*, the objectivity of these sources being seldom challenged.[5] However, the universally beneficial effects of registration have since been queried, firstly by Bob Little, who argued from oral sources that the Act's requirements led to the loss of safe and well-respected local midwives from working-class communities,[6] and secondly by Brooke Heagerty, who claimed that the intention of the registration movement, 'an organised minority of socially influential aristocratic and middle class women', was to create a new profession with themselves as its elite.[7] Their innovative work encouraged investigation of actual nineteenth-century midwifery practice, drawing on previously unexplored sources. Census and Post Office Directory entries have been combined to create a picture of nurses and midwives as businesswomen;[8] and analyses of hospital and charity casebooks have argued that their midwives were reliable, safe and respected by the institution's doctors,[9] although local authority material gives a less positive impression.[10] More attention has also been paid to national differences.[11]

Thus the last 25 years have seen the emergence of a more complex picture of midwifery in Britain in the nineteenth and early twentieth centuries. This chapter will explore these complexities, dividing the period into three sections: 1800–60, 1860–1902 and 1902–20.

In Whom 'the community [has] the fullest confidence': Midwives, 1800–60

Between 1800 and 1860 Britain became increasingly industrialized, with implications for the work of midwives. However, much of the intellectual structure that supported later debates about midwifery in industrial society was not yet in place. Insofar as there was interest in women's health, it was thought that working-class women were able to cope with hard work and poor diet, unlike middle-class women who required medical supervision.[12] Midwifery occupied debatable ground: seen by the medical elite as a manual occupation 'foreign to the habits of Gentlemen of enlarged academical education', it was nevertheless considered to be the key to successful general practice.[13] Despite the disdain of the profession's leaders, male midwifery practice continued to expand throughout the century, threatening to eclipse that of the midwife, and largely replacing her as birth attendant of choice among the middle and wealthier classes. Nonetheless, medical interest in the topic was limited; in 1848 there were only four references to midwifery in the *British Medical Journal*; 40 years later, in 1889, there were 52. James Young Simpson, Professor of Midwifery at Edinburgh University, felt compelled to begin each annual lecture course by defending his subject and its social value in terms of lives saved; despite his application of the anaesthetic effects of chloroform to childbirth in 1847, he emphasized the role of nature and discouraged unnecessary intervention. Infant health was not a national concern. Before the introduction of vital registration in 1837 (1855 in Scotland), births and deaths might go unrecorded, while the collection of medical statistics (crucial for assessing the effectiveness of care and carers) was unusual and small-scale.[14]

Little is known about the number of midwives. The 1841 census recorded 676 midwives in England and Wales (with a population of 15,911,757), and 641 in Scotland (with a population of 2,620,184). Ten years later, 2,067 midwives were recorded in England and Wales, and 815 in Scotland.[15] The apparent substantial increase between 1841 and 1851 in England and Wales and the ratio of one midwife to approximately 4,000 people in Scotland together suggest that these were not accurate records. It is likely that census enumerators did not recognize midwifery's part-time nature, particularly in thinly populated areas, and therefore did not count all midwives in practice. For example, Ann Wood, one of four midwives in Cullen in whom the community had 'the fullest confidence', combined 18 years of part-time midwifery practice with keeping a public house with her husband.[16] Even in 1904 a letter to *Nursing Notes* described 'two little country parishes . . . straggling . . . remote', averaging 27 births a year, attended by two elderly midwives but where no younger woman could afford to work.[17] The restrictions on sick nursing and laying out the dead which would result from the first Midwives' Act in 1902 were seen as interfering with necessary supplementary income.[18]

There is equally limited evidence for where midwives practised, but they were apparently widespread. Margaret Robertson (trained at the Edinburgh Royal Maternity Hospital (ERMH) in 1848) practised in Arbroath before emigrating to New Zealand in 1863, taking with her a testimonial from a local doctor: 'I . . . meet her occasionally in a professional way. From what I know of her . . . she is worthy of confidence and do recommend her accordingly';[19] in 1851 the census recorded 52 midwives in Aberdeen, and 40 in Edinburgh and Leith.[20] South of the border, between 1842 and 1852, *Provincial Medical Journal* correspondents referred to midwives in Wales, Rochdale, Manchester, Salford, Droitwich, Bridgewater, Swaffham and Hampshire, suggesting a reasonable spread. Royal Maternity Charity (RMC) midwives covered much of central London.

Although the elderly midwife would later be caricatured, Mrs Cowper's ever-expanding practice suggests that age and experience were greatly valued by clients. Similarly, Dr Bishop, called to attend a cross birth (shoulder presentation), described the primary attendant, 'an old midwife . . . . upwards of eighty years of age', in mainly positive terms. 'Her faculties were clear and good, and she often boasted to me of having "followed the art" . . . and having attended several hundred cases.'[21] Nevertheless, midwives were undoubtedly an ageing population, with the implication of an occupation in decline. In 1851 in Edinburgh, 12 midwives (one-third of the sample) were less than 45 years old, but by 1861 only two were. In the same year 31 per cent of the 492 midwives recorded in the Irish census were over 60.[22] Two-thirds of the Edinburgh group were widowed,[23] though, in an age of common and fatal infections and industrial accidents, widowhood did not necessarily equal age. Margaret Bethune, for example, was widowed at 32 by a mining accident and, after some training in Edinburgh, supported her two children and elderly mother by working as a midwife in Lower Largo, Fife.[24]

Most midwives worked independently, combining private cases with work for local charities, as RMC midwives did.[25] Poor Law Unions apparently preferred to 'sanction the employment of very ignorant midwives' to deliver parturient paupers, rather than the more expensive Medical Officer.[26] In 1847–8, Mrs Elizabeth Mate, the Islington Union midwife, averaged 260 Poor Law deliveries a year, earning £65 from these alone.[27] Mrs Eaves was paid 3s 6d for 'workhouse' births, and also attended deliveries for the Coventry Ladies Lying-in Charity, in addition to private cases. In contrast, Mrs Johnston, 'a bred midwife [who had] . . . delivered patients to the extent of hundreds', and Matron to the ERMH, was salaried. Her role included 'teach[ing] the midwives and nurses', plus responsibility for the house-keeping and discipline of the Hospital.[28] Increasingly, many women combined midwifery with monthly nursing, providing private live-in intra- and postnatal care of mother and baby under medical supervision, the doctor being responsible for the delivery, a trend that had started in the previous century.[29]

Although doctors were clearly beginning to feel the economic competition,[30] the implication of much contemporary material was that midwives were welcome and reliable colleagues. Simpson praised their low maternal mortality rates;[31] others their intelligence and experience.[32] In Wales, Dr Coats of Sirhowy and Dr Hinton of Blaina Ironworks both enjoyed a good relationship with local midwives, only being called to emergency cases.[33] Although some correspondents criticized midwives, the medical journals themselves were more concerned with the deficiencies of men-midwives, the lurid nature of such cases increasing as the Medical Registration Act approached.[34]

Mrs Cowper was possibly unusual in learning through formal lectures and practice. Some midwives learned 'traditionally', by personal experience of birth, combined with accompanying an experienced midwife. This apprenticeship approach to training is evident in the records, with family connections sometimes apparent. For example, Mrs Bradley Senior and Mrs Bradley practised in 1820s Manchester, with their shared name suggesting that they were mother- and daughter-in-law.[35] A doctor or lying-in charity might set up a short training course; some offered free training in exchange for a period of work. Although the standards of such courses were later criticized, there is little objective evidence of poor quality. In 1826 the Aberdeen Medico-Chirurgical Society appointed 'a committee to examine and grant certificates to midwives...to increase the[ir] respectability...and give the public additional confidence in their skill'. Aspiring midwives were examined in their knowledge of pelvic anatomy, management of labour, diseases of pregnancy and the puerperium, infant care, therapeutic bleeding and catheter use. This scheme was popular, but ceased in 1831, though not through lack of support. In that year five midwives from Aberdeen and twelve from country parishes received certificates.[36] Midwives were examined and licensed by the Faculty of Physicians and Surgeons of Glasgow from 1740 until the 1820s; thereafter voluntary training was associated with the city's maternity hospital.[37] In London, training was available at the British Lying-In and City of London Hospitals, and in 1830 the British Ladies Lying-In Institution, intended to provide well-trained midwives for both private practice among the rich and charity work, was founded under the patronage of the Duchess of Kent. Initially instruction was given by its 'Consulting Midwife', Mrs C. M. Beale, but by 1858 she had been replaced by a surgeon-accoucheur.[38] Training had been available at the Rotunda in Dublin since the mid-eighteenth century; unusually lasting six months, it prepared women for employment as parish midwives under the Irish Poor Law.[39]

The content of midwifery training is harder to reconstruct. Theoretical lecture courses similar to that attended by Mrs Cowper continued in Edinburgh. In 1850, 25 midwives attended the ERMH in conjunction with a lecture course, typically being present at 6 deliveries and gaining minimal exposure to obstetric emergencies. This compared poorly with the experience of male students at the same hospital, who combined a daily lecture on midwifery with copious unsupervised practical experience, although it can be suggested that the women had prior experience which made practical training less important.[40]

Mrs Bethune's casebook shows she was able to identify cases where medical aid was necessary. She never lost a mother, while the number of repeat cases and, later, deliveries of 'her' babies suggest she was greatly respected locally.[41] Other midwives were also capable of dealing successfully and resourcefully with emergencies; in 1846 'Mrs Baker, a midwife' dealt with haemorrhage until medical aid arrived by applying 'cold wet cloths ... to the [patient's] abdomen'.[42] Similarly, in 1855 when 'the placenta did not come away immediately, the midwife got her [patient] out of bed, and put her in the erect position, to blow in a bottle, which brought the placenta away without any interference'.[43]

Towards Registration: Midwifery, 1860–1902

The second half of the nineteenth century saw many changes in medicine and society. Philanthropic concern for the poor became more organized, and anxiety grew for the survival and health firstly of infants,[44] and then of their mothers, charitable ladies arguing their shared gender gave them insight into the lives of poor women. Medically, the discovery and application of antisepsis simultaneously offered a means to prevent infection and the implication of improper treatment by any attendant if infection arose,[45] while the subsequent rise of a more interventionist approach to obstetrics began to divide it from midwifery.[46] Many actual and proposed changes in British midwifery in this period were associated with the passing of the Medical Registration Act in 1858 and its amendment in 1886. Like the Midwives' Act to come, its purpose was to limit the appropriate title to holders of certain qualifications (including long practice). However, midwifery continued to be viewed with suspicion by the medical elite, and initially a midwifery qualification was unnecessary for registration. This stimulated both debates about the nature of midwifery practice and experiments in training.

Two new schools for midwives were founded, although ultimately neither showed much awareness of the realities of contemporary practice. The first was Florence Nightingale's training school at King's College Hospital, opened in 1862 but closed five years later due to the high incidence of puerperal fever deaths.[47] This provided six months' training to sponsored village 'midwifery nurses'. By the time she published her *Notes on Lying-In Institutions* in 1871, Nightingale not only had used an analysis of its failure to postulate what a future maternity hospital should be like but had also done the same for midwifery training, typically by comparison (and not to its advantage) with that currently offered by the second institution, the Ladies' Medical College.

Opened in 1864, with the initial intention of providing well-trained midwives but the ultimate goal of training women for the medical profession, the Ladies' Medical College was the creation of the incongruously named all-male Female Medical Society. The main driver behind its foundation and organization was Society-member Dr James Edmunds (early supporter of Semmelweis, advocate of single-purpose childbirth attendants and a former RMC district surgeon): in fact the College was based in his London home. It offered a longer training to atypical midwife trainees, including already-practising midwives, matrons, missionaries and philanthropic amateurs. Its course incorporated lectures by an obstetrician 'during two winter sessions' with time spent 'during the intervening summer' at a Lying-in Hospital or maternity charity, 'with personal attendance upon at least *twenty-five* deliveries'. This was the aspect criticized by Nightingale, who felt that 25 cases offered only a small chance of seeing any emergencies, in comparison with the three years of experience potentially offered to medical students.[48] She now advocated 'not less than two years' of training to produce 'real physician accoucheuses . . . to attend and be consulted in all deliveries, abnormal as well as normal, in diseases of women and children', in a single-function hospital.[49] Although successful in its short life (in 1867 it claimed 50 enrolments), the College, like Nightingale's unrealized lying-in institution, was too radical in its expectation of commitment of time and money to fit comfortably in British midwifery at the time. Its survival was not helped by Edmunds' abrasive nature, and it closed in 1872.[50]

However, a number of less contentious, more successful local training schemes were begun at this period 'in London, Manchester, and other large towns by the medical officers connected with lying-in hospitals'.[51] For example, training in Sheffield, begun around 1878, was associated with the Jessop Hospital for Women, and trainees, unusually funded by the Hospital, were expected to continue to work for it on a case-by-case basis once trained. As pupils, they attended at least 30 labours, and were competent to identify complications requiring medical aid.[52] By 1875 Manchester had a body of trained midwives, provided with 'difficult case' cards to return to the hospital when help was needed.[53] In Edinburgh in 1870 there were again 25 pupil midwives at the ERMH, typically attending ten cases each during their three months' stay. In addition to theoretical lectures (which in some instances were shared with medical students),[54] within the Hospital they watched the medical management of more difficult cases, including manipulative deliveries and haemorrhage.[55] In Ireland, a course for army midwives was begun in 1868 at Sir Patrick Duns Hospital, Dublin. Four years later, 136 midwives had been trained. Again, the course was free, but the women were expected to be educated, and of good character and conduct. In their six-month training they delivered between 30 and 70 cases, and heard lectures on midwifery and the 'Laws of Health and Climate'.[56]

There was little change in the demographic profile of women recruited. The 17 midwives identified in the 1881 census in Sheffield, who included those trained at the Jessop, were aged between 44 and 63, of working-class origin and typically widowed.[57] The five pupils at the ERMH on census night in 1871 were aged from 24 to 49; three were married, one single and one widowed. Even 20 years later, when a new matron began a Register of midwife pupils, there had been little change. Several women were sent by their local landowner, a form of patronage in use since the eighteenth century; widows were prominent, if not predominant; origins were often working class.[58]

A midwife trained at this period in Edinburgh described herself thus:

> I have been in practice in the Braes of Lochaber for 40 years. I was trained by Dr Matthews Duncan. I was taught by him to exercise patience and never to get flustered or to hurry. I have never had a death at a confinement. The cases were mostly 'natural.' Few required a doctor. I judged by experience when to send for him.[59]

Complaints about such practitioners were rare: giving evidence to the Select Committee in 1892, Dr Napier was enthusiastic.[60] More practically, the institutions that trained such midwives made a favourable impression on the local maternal mortality rate.[61]

However, any provincial progress was not reflected in the London Obstetrical Society (LOS) survey of midwives and their practice carried out in 1869. The Society had been formed following the Medical Act, with the aim of excluding or controlling 'dubious' practitioners, particularly midwives. It too had no idea of the number of midwives or the extent of their practice, and in 1869 sent out a questionnaire to Society members. Doctors were asked of their locality '[w]hat proportion of births is attended by medical men and by midwives' and whether the midwives were 'instructed'. Respondents gave a very variable picture:

> Among the poor population of villages a large proportion, varying from thirty to ninety per cent, is attended by midwives. In the small non-manufacturing towns ... attendance by midwives prevails to a much less extent.... In the large provincial towns, and especially in large manufacturing towns, attendance by midwives among the labouring population occurs in almost as large proportion as in the agricultural villages.

In 'the east' of London, 30–50 per cent of 'the poor' were attended by midwives, yet 'in the west' only 2 per cent were.[62]

Few doctors believed their local midwives had had any instruction.

> Answers in the negative have been received from all parts of the country. From several districts the replies indicate not merely a want of any special education, but gross ignorance and incompetence, and a complete inability to contend with any difficulty that may occur. In London ... many women practis[e] midwifery who have

received . . . instruction at various institutions, but these, although fairly competent in ordinary cases, are also quite unequal to any of the emergencies of obstetrics.[63]

It is difficult to interpret the survey findings. Later criticisms from doctors that midwives often waited until a complication was irrefutable before calling for help can be interpreted as resulting from the growing gap between the attitudes of doctors and midwives, whereby doctors began increasingly to anticipate problems, while midwives retained their previous confidence in nature.[64] However, the survey criticisms precede this period, suggesting that they may be justified. It is also the case that the data and methodology of the survey are dubious (even the Society President, Dr Grailly Hewitt, questioned them when giving his evidence to the Select Committee 20 years later):[65] it was nonetheless very influential.

The LOS resolved to improve midwifery practice, and established a diploma for those with the 'minimum amount of knowledge which an ordinary midwife should have . . . it is hoped that the distinction [conferred by possession of a certificate] will induce midwives to seek the instruction necessary to obtain it'.[66] Although criticized as London-centric even by contemporaries,[67] the LOS examination became the gold standard for midwifery in the last quarter of the century. In August 1891 the written paper asked for a description of the passage of the foetal head through the pelvis in a posterior position; the management of labour following spontaneous rupture of membranes resulting in a foot visible at the vulva; knowledge of the type and concentration of antiseptics for specific tasks; and the advice to be given on establishing breastfeeding. Fifty-five entrants passed, 17 trained outwith London. Between 1872 and 1891, over 1,000 women received the LOS diploma.[68] The LOS also raised the question of registration, their initial suggestions reflecting typical practice by defining midwifery in terms of medical assistance and domestic help. Registered midwives were to relieve the burden on doctors by attending natural labours among the poor, and that on new mothers by helping with housework. Despite the more extensive training offered by the Ladies' Medical College, there was to be only one (basic) grade of practitioner.[69]

In 1881 registration was taken up by a new organization, the Matron's Aid or Trained Midwives' Registration Society (from 1886, the Midwives' Institute). Its founders represented a new type of midwife. Mainly single women from upper middle-class families, like

Mrs Stephens, they had undergone post-Nightingale nurse training before gaining the LOS diploma.[70] Unlike her, they had family connections among the medical and charitable elite, and embraced midwifery as a philanthropic cause rather than a source of necessary income.[71] They considered LOS leaders their social equals, and they were able to harness elected politicians and new women's pressure groups to their cause[72] and had the funds to set up a journal to publicize and reinforce their views among their membership.[73] Nonetheless, their knowledge of the actual practice of midwifery in Britain was dubious – the statistics used in the Society's prospectus came from the LOS survey, and its sweeping assertions that there was a desperate need for 'an increase in the number of trained and licensed midwives . . . [that in 1881] only 80 women hold a certificate of any value' can certainly be questioned.[74] Only in 1900 did the Institute enquire into the actual numbers, employment and suitability for further education of rural midwives.[75] They felt little *esprit de corps*, being as ready as medical correspondents to raise the spectres of Sarah Gamp or Mother Midnight (an equally fictional midwife, bawd and brothel-keeper), and to blame practising midwives for failure to resuscitate the newborn, for the spread of ophthalmia neonatorum (highly contagious eye infection of the newborn) and for procuring abortions.[76]

Nonetheless, their independence enabled the Midwives' Institute to withstand the attacks which followed the 1886 Medical Act, which, for the first time, made knowledge of midwifery necessary for qualification as a doctor. As a result, medical schools found themselves struggling to provide students with sufficient maternity cases,[77] and casting greedy glances towards those poor women delivered by midwives. The General Medical Council (GMC) withdrew its previous support for midwife registration, and throughout the 1890s female midwifery was subject to spiteful attacks. For example, the LOS was forced to alter the wording of its certificate, and others were completely withdrawn, as being 'colourable imitation[s]' of a medical diploma.[78] Many general practitioners (GPs), nervous at the increased competition, became particularly aggressive towards trained midwives.[79]

This new antagonism led to the establishment of a Select Committee to enquire into the need for registration. Hearing evidence over two years, it concluded that

> a serious amount of suffering and permanent injury to women and children is caused from the inefficiency and want of skill of many of the

women practising as midwives, without proper training or qualification. [Yet] ... amongst the poor and working classes ... the services of properly trained midwives have been eminently successful [and]. ... are a necessity.[80]

Despite these findings, medical opposition to midwifery registration continued. Between 1895 and 1900 there were four failed attempts, before, in 1902, the Midwives' Act (England and Wales) was passed.

Even before the Act, the long years of campaigning influenced midwives' training and practice. The key role possession of the LOS certificate would play in registration became widely recognized, and many more candidates took the examination: in June 1895, 90 women passed; five years later, 221 did so. Mrs Layton, a midwife from Cricklewood, was not among them. Coached by the doctor with whom she worked (and discouraged by him from seeking hospital training), when faced with a 'written examination ... at 9 p.m., in a closely packed room [with] two hours to answer the questions, and a fortnight later an oral examination', she, and 'about 130' others, failed.[81]

Implementing the Midwives Acts, 1902–20

The 1902 Midwives' Act (England and Wales) limited certification to women who held midwifery certificates from the LOS, or from four named Irish institutions or 'such other certificate as may be approved', and to those women who had been in *bona fide* practice for at least one year before the passing of the Act, and were of 'good character'. Two years were allowed for registration. After 1 April 1905, the title of midwife was to be limited to those certified under the Act; thereafter certification would follow successful examination. From 1910, no uncertified woman was to practise 'habitually and for gain', unless 'under the direction of a qualified medical practitioner' (this was to protect monthly nurses).[82] Controlled at local level by a local supervising authority (LSA), appointed by the county or borough council, midwives would be governed nationally by the Central Midwives' Board (CMB). This consisted of four medical practitioners, who were appointed by the two Royal Colleges, the Society of Apothecaries and the Midwives' Institute; single representatives from the County Councils, the Queen Victoria Jubilee Institute and the Royal British Nurses Association; and two Privy Council appointees, one to be a woman. No midwife sat on the new profession's governing body by right, although the first three female CMB members were all qualified midwives. This omission has been interpreted variously as a reflection of the social links between the midwifery elite and the medical profession, and as the price paid for success. Nonetheless, the Institute's President, Jane Wilson, resigned from the Board in protest.[83] Only in 1920 was the need for a midwife member recognized.

As a result of the Act, for the first time there was an accurate record of the number of midwives in England and Wales. By April 1905, the Roll contained 22,308 names: 7,465 LOS diplomates, 2,322 with recognized hospital certificates, and 12,521 in *bona fide* practice.[84] Nonetheless, this may still not be an accurate reflection of actual practice. Some certificate holders enrolled while not working as midwives; others registered by circuitous routes. Miss Lucretia Hewitt, for example, trained in Edinburgh and working as a midwife and monthly nurse in Scotland (not covered by the Act), nevertheless took advantage of the CMB's recognition of the ERMH as a training centre in 1904 to enrol.[85] The Act implied that the mechanism of supervision was already in place, but this was far from the case. Reports in *Nursing Notes* suggest that only in 1904 were councils becoming organized to provide this.[86] In 1905 the journal regretted that six counties which had no Medical Officer of Health (MOH) had delegated their powers under the Midwives' Act to 'local bodies', suspecting that it would be 'less uniformly administered'. Some kept their powers in the hands of council members of Public Health or Sanitary Committees; others created special Midwives' Act Committees, with 'co-opted ladies'. By January 1905, 34 Inspectors of Midwives had been appointed.[87]

The actions of LSAs have been interpreted as either improving the standards of the profession, or using intimidation to dismantle 'the intricate network of working-class relationships'.[88] However, a recent analysis of their work in Bradford has taken at face-value the claim of the Institute that its primary aim was protection for mothers, and has concentrated on the benefits for maternal health. Inspectors of Midwives in the city produced a rapid improvement in the quality of midwifery care and in outcomes for mothers and infants. Nonetheless, they did not harass 'their' midwives, but made their lives easier, providing postage-paid birth notification forms and encouraging the city fathers' plan for a savings scheme to help poor mothers meet their delivery costs.[89] Similarly, in Manchester, the efficient supervision and education policy of its Inspector, Dr Merry Smith, produced a swift improvement in the professionalism of the city's midwives.[90] Following a lecture course in 1906, Sheffield's MOH looked to the city's midwives to provide new mothers with approved advice on hygiene and infant feeding.[91] However, inspection may have brought little immediate change outside conurbations. In Wales, Nurse Davies, a devout Methodist, continued to practise as she had been taught by her mother to the hour of her death, placing her faith in herbal tonics and strict cleanliness.[92] Although chronologically later, an ethnographic exploration of twentieth-century childbirth in rural Ulster between 1935 and 1970 also found little alteration in childbirth customs and behaviour until hospitalization became common.[93]

The restrictions of the CMB and the Midwives' Institute were not wholly unopposed, implying tensions between London-based and provincial organizations. Even before the Act was passed, the Manchester Midwives Society had, in 1899, questioned the wisdom of registration under medical control.[94] The knowledge and standards of Manchester's trained midwives were attacked at a Queen Victoria Jubilee Nurses Institute conference in 1904, when district nurses specifically accused 'those who have grand brass plates on their door testifying that they have received a diploma from one of the hospitals' of poor standards of care, failure to grasp elementary hygiene and illiteracy, criticizing the short length of their training and recommending additional initial nurse training.[95] A reasoned response from Manchester appeared in the next edition of *Nursing Notes*, pointing out that as Institute district nurses refused to attend cases with local midwives they could not know directly how well or badly they cared for patients; that a written examination had always been required as part of local training; and that while only 'District Hospital' midwives were required to use antiseptics under hospital rules, for all midwives 'it pays us to do our duty' with regard to hygiene and cleanliness of mother and baby. The patronizing tone of the accompanying comments in *Nursing Notes* ('no one supposes there are no efficient midwives in the town') suggests an element of class as well as professional antagonism in this incident.[96] Two new organizations were founded, whose membership grew rapidly in the north: the British Union of Midwives (supported by the Women's Trade Union League) and the National Association of Midwives. They asserted that, as midwives had not been in association when the Act was passed, the Institute had 'no moral right to the title which it assume[d]'. They believed practising midwives knew best for their profession, and did 'not need to be fussed over and patronized. They [were] tired of "charity-mongers"; they [were] sick of being "bossed"'. However, although the Union and the National Association continued to promote direct representation of rank-and-file midwives and the creation of a state maternity service until 1914, both organizations effectively faded after the failure of the 1910 Departmental Committee to make any major changes to the Midwives' Act, and the merger of their journal, the *Midwives Record*, with *Nurses' Own Magazine*.[97]

The ERMH Nurses' Register suggests that the Act resulted in changes to the type of women becoming midwives: they were younger (half of the 1912 intake was under 30), almost all were single and over half had had previous nursing experience and took the shorter (four-month) training. Not all sat the CMB examination (travelling to Newcastle to do so), but those who did were typically nurse-trained and single, with an average age of 31.[98] However, the same Registers indicate some reversion to recruiting non-nurse widows during the First World War. Interestingly, a number of sources suggest the 'new midwife' was less welcome to patients than the old.[99]

The academic knowledge required for midwifery practice was now defined by the CMB, and included elementary pelvic anatomy, pregnancy and its complications, the mechanism, management and course of natural labour, the signs of abnormal labour, the immediate treatment of obstetric emergencies until the arrival of medical aid, the puerperal care of mother and child, and the use of thermometer and catheter. Practical training was to include 20 cases of 'personal delivery'. Practice was limited to normal labour, including uncomplicated breech presentation; medical aid was required for all other cases. Nonetheless, the Act had not addressed the issue of payment for such aid, and this, plus the interpretation that calling for aid implied the midwife controlled the doctor, continued to be an issue.[100] When the Act was passed in 1916 in Scotland, it required the costs of such calls to be borne by the local authority.

Scotland had initially been excluded from the Act because it would have required separate legislation, and it was felt that, with a longer tradition of medical education in midwifery, the independent midwife was an anachronism who would fade away. Three factors increased the demand for an equivalent act. A high rate of puerperal infection was associated with unregulated midwifery practice; changes in local authority powers made the adoption of English legislation in Scotland possible; and by 1915 the absence of many medical practitioners on war service led to an increased demand for competent midwives in Scotland. The Midwives Scotland Act received Royal Assent in December 1915 and came into force on 1 January 1916.[101]

Ireland had similarly been excluded; in 1902 the interest of its Royal College was largely limited to defending Irish midwifery certificates. However, by the time of the Act's review in 1910, the role of the midwife as the attendant for 'the poorer classes in the case of normal childbirth' was largely accepted.[102] Nonetheless, extension of the Act was not considered a priority, partly because Poor Law Unions already had considerable power in employing midwives. However, the passage of the Act in Scotland led to increased pressure, and in November 1917 an Irish Midwives' Bill was introduced to the House of Commons. By February 1918 the Bill was awaiting Royal Assent; in May the medical representatives, who again dominated the Board, were being elected.[103]

Conclusion

The nineteenth century saw the beginning of the transition of British midwifery from local community-based women, who mainly learnt their craft via apprenticeship and whose skills were of variable quality, to regulated and trained professionals, whose practice was tightly defined and monitored. By 1920 the role of the midwife in normal labour and birth was enshrined in legislation in all the countries of Britain, but her earlier autonomy is likely to have been compromised by the limitations imposed by the various Midwifery Acts, on which doctors exerted considerable influence. The nature of her work, at this time still largely domiciliary and therefore isolated, imposed further limitations. Although the devolved nature of LSAs has exposed them to criticism of having private agendas rather than a common standard, their often-supportive role in the professional development of midwives should be recognized, when the Midwives' Institute was initially slow to expand outwith the London area and was widely perceived as having little in common with ordinary practitioners.

Whereas, at the beginning of the period covered by this chapter, midwifery had been largely an occupation for women drawn from the local community, whose working-class origin reflected Victorian ideas of female employment and whose frequently widowed status illustrated their own lack of support, by the end it was increasingly a profession for previously nurse-trained single women of wider social origins, in this both reflecting and contributing to the growing medicalization of childbirth. Such a change in social background weakened the former close relationship between practitioner and patient; it is doubtful whether it strengthened that between doctor and midwife.

Acknowledgements

I would like to thank Susan McGann, Fiona Bourne and Anne Cameron of the RCN Archives, the staff of Lothian Health Services Archive, the Inter-Library Loan Services of Edinburgh and Southampton Universities for their help, and Professors Rosemary Mander and Roger Davidson for their advice and support.

Notes

1. Royal College of Physicians of Edinburgh [RCPEd.], Christian Cowper, Midwifery Book, Jan 1786–1843.
2. *The Midwives Register: Mary Eaves, Midwife of Spon End, Coventry, 1847–1875*, transcribed by B. Wishart (Coventry: Coventry Family History Society, 2000).
3. B. Cowell and D. Wainwright, *Behind the Blue Door: The History of the Royal College of Midwives, 1881–1981* (London: Baillière Tindall, 1981) pp. 40–1.
4. *Nursing Notes*, 7 (1894) 41–2.
5. See, in particular, Cowell and Wainwright, *Blue Door*; J. Towler and J. Bramall, *Midwives in History and Society* (London: Croom Helm, 1986); J. Ferlie, 'A Historical Survey of Midwifery in Scotland', *International Journal of Nursing Studies*, 1 (1963–64) 125–9; and the immensely detailed (and feminist) J. Donnison, *Midwives and Medical Men: A History of the Struggle for the Control of Childbirth*, 2nd edn (London: Historical Publications, 1988).
6. B. Little, ' "Go Seek Mrs. Dawson – She'll Know What to Do": The Demise of the Working-Class Nurse/Midwife in the Early Twentieth Century', Essex University, MA thesis (1983).
7. B. V. Heagerty, 'Class, Gender and Professionalization: The Struggle for British Midwifery 1900–36', Michigan State University, PhD thesis (1990) pp. ii–iii; B. V. Heagerty, 'Willing Handmaidens of Science? The Struggle over the New Midwife in Early Twentieth-Century England', in M. J. Kirkham and E. R. Perkins (eds), *Reflections on Midwifery* (London: Baillière Tindall, 1997) pp. 70–95. For a more measured view, see J. Hannam, 'Rosalind Paget: The Midwife, the Women's Movement and Reform before 1914', in H. Marland and A. M. Rafferty (eds), *Midwives, Society and Childbirth: Debates and Controversies in the Modern Period* (London: Routledge, 1997) pp. 81–101.

8. B. E. Mortimer, 'The Nurse in Edinburgh c.1760–1860: The Impact of Commerce and Professionalisation', Edinburgh University, PhD thesis (2002); B.E. Mortimer, 'Independent Women: Domiciliary Nurses in Mid-Nineteenth-Century Edinburgh', in A. M. Rafferty, J. Robinson and R. Elkan (eds), *Nursing History and the Politics of Welfare* (London: Routledge, 1997) pp. 132–49.

9. S. A. Seligman, 'The Royal Maternity Charity: The First Hundred Years', *Medical History*, 24:4 (1980) 403–18; C. Stephenson, 'The Voluntary Maternity Hospital: A Social History of Provincial Institutions', Warwick University, PhD thesis (1993); T. McIntosh, 'A Price Must Be Paid for Motherhood: The Experience of Maternity in Sheffield, 1879–1939', Sheffield University, PhD thesis (1997); T. McIntosh, 'Profession, Skill or Domestic Duty? Midwifery in Sheffield, 1881–1936', *Social History of Medicine*, 11:3 (1998) 403–20; A. M. Nuttall, 'A Preliminary Survey of Midwifery Training in Edinburgh, 1844 to 1870', *International History of Nursing Journal*, 4 (1998–99) 4–14; A. M. Nuttall, 'The Edinburgh Royal Maternity Hospital and the Medicalisation of Childbirth in Edinburgh 1844–1914: A Casebook-Centred Perspective', Edinburgh University, PhD thesis (2003).

10. J. Mottram, 'State Control in Local Context: Public Health and Midwife Regulation in Manchester, 1900–1914', in Marland and Rafferty (eds), *Midwives*, pp. 134–52; P. Dale and K. Fisher, 'Implementing the 1902 Midwives Act: Assessing Problems, Developing Services and Creating a New Role for a Variety of Female Practitioners', *Women's History Review*, 18:3 (2009) 427–52.

11. L. Reid, 'Scottish Midwives (1916–1983): The Central Midwives Board for Scotland and Practising Midwives', Glasgow University, PhD thesis, 2003; L. Reid, *Midwifery in Scotland: A History* (Erskine: Scottish History Press, 2011); A. McMahon, 'Regulating Midwives: The Role of the Royal College of Physicians of Ireland', in G. M. Fealy (ed.), *Care to Remember: Nursing and Midwifery in Ireland* (Cork: Mercier Press, 2005) pp. 158–71.

12. J. Bedford, 'Who Should Deliver Babies? Models of Nature and the Midwifery Debate in England c.1800–c.1886', London University, PhD thesis (1995) pp. 25–6.

13. Sir Henry Halford, President of the Royal College of Physicians, cited in Donnison, *Midwives*, p. 57. See also I. Loudon, *Medical Care and the General Practitioner 1750–1850* (Oxford: Clarendon Press, 1986); Bedford, 'Who Should Deliver Babies?', pp. 115, 124–7.

14. J. M Eyler, *Victorian Social Medicine: The Ideas and Methods of William Farr* (Baltimore and London: The Johns Hopkins University Press, 1979) pp. 37–47; I. Loudon, *Death in Childbirth: An International Study of Maternal Care and Maternal Mortality, 1800–1950* (Oxford: Clarendon Press, 1992) pp. 23–5. Loudon observes that the initial

1837 Act placed the burden of registering both births and deaths (his principal focus) on the local registrar; its revision in 1874 (the Births and Deaths Registration Act, 1974) shifted that burden to the parents or nearest relative. Acquisition of accurate data on labour and delivery was Simpson's principal motive for creating the detailed casebooks of the ERMH. See Nuttall, 'Edinburgh Royal Maternity Hospital', pp. 19–21. Occasionally correspondents to medical journals submitted their midwifery practice statistics; others claimed to keep none. See, for example, *Provincial Medical Journal* (10 June 1846) 261–3; *British Medical Journal* (2 April 1864) 367–8.

15. Mortimer, 'Nurse', p. 90.

16. Mrs Wood, 'a person of respectable family, of steady integrity, of circumspect behaviour, of thorough veracity', trained in Aberdeen in 1849, and averaged 35–40 deliveries annually. See J. Wilson, *Truth: A Libel by Law. The Evidence of Sir J. Y. Simpson, Bart., M.D., and Others, in the Case of Sharp versus Wilson, with correspondence* (Edinburgh: Henry Robinson, 1869) pp. 63, 92.

17. *Nursing Notes*, 16 (1904) 108.

18. *Nursing Notes*, 17 (1905) 87.

19. Midwifery Papers of Mrs Margaret Robertson (photocopies), accessed 1996–97, but now mislaid within the collections (Edinburgh University Library [EUL], Lothian Health Services Archive [LHSA], LHB MAC GD 1/27/1-3).

20. Mortimer, 'Nurse', p. 117.

21. *Provincial Medical and Surgical Journal* (23 April 1852) 208–9. However, less positively, Bishop then speculated that '[w]e may therefore fairly infer she has deprived the local medical officer of many hundred pounds'. For a contrasting case and medical attitude, see *Association Medical Journal* (25 May 1855) 485–6.

22. J. A Bergin, 'Childbirth and Midwifery in Ireland, c.1745–c.1900', in E. Farrell (ed.), *'She said she was in the family way:' Pregnancy and Infancy in Modern Ireland* (London: Institute of Historical Research) (April 2012).

23. Mortimer, 'Nurse', p. 122.

24. Mortimer, 'Nurse', pp. 198–220.

25. See also *Association Medical Journal* (2 February 1856) 85–6; (15 March 1856) 209–10.

26. *Association Medical Journal* (2 February 1856) 95.

27. Donnison, *Midwives*, pp. 69, 218, Note 82.

28. EUL, LHSA, Edinburgh Royal Maternity Hospital [ERMH], Directors' Minutes, LHB 3/1/2, p. 100. 'Bred' means trained.

29. Mortimer, 'Independent Women', pp. 137–9.

30. See Notes 21 and 25.

31. J.Y. Simpson, *Two Letters to Dr. Collins, President of the King and Queen's College of Physicians of Ireland etc. I. On the Duration of Labour as a Cause of Mortality and Danger to Mother and Child. II. On the Obstetrical Statistics of the Dublin Hospital* (Edinburgh: Sutherland and Knox, 1848) p. 16.

32. *Association Medical Journal* (10 May 1856) 385; (2 March 1855) 203–4.

33. *Association Medical Journal* (20 July 1855) 679–80; (1 September 1854) 792.

34. See, for example, *British Medical Journal* (18 April 1857) 323–4; (25 April 1857) 345–6.

35. *Association Medical Journal* (2 February 1856) 85; (10 May 1856) 382. See also *British Medical Journal* (6 May 1865) 459 for a mother and daughter in practice in Westminster.

36. J. Jenkinson, *Scottish Medical Societies* (Edinburgh: Edinburgh University Press, 1993) pp. 82–3; G. P. Milne, 'A History of Midwifery in Eighteenth, Nineteenth and Early Twentieth Century Aberdeen', *Medical History*, 22 (1978) 205–6.

37. D. A. Dow, *The Rottenrow* (Carnforth: The Parthenon Press, 1984).

38. Donnison, *Midwives*, pp. 62–3.

39. Donnison, *Midwives*, pp. 77, 96; I. C. Ross, *Public Virtue, Public Love: The Early Years of the Dublin Lying-in Hospital – the Rotunda* (Dublin: O'Brien Press, 1986) pp. 9–52. However, numbers were small: Bergin reports that only 14–18 midwives a year graduated from the Rotunda and Coombe Hospitals together (Bergin, 'Childbirth').

40. Nuttall, 'Edinburgh Royal Maternity Hospital', pp. 250–3.

41. Mortimer, 'Nurse', pp. 208–19.

42. *Provincial Medical and Surgical Journal* (8 April 1846) 162–3.

43. *Association Medical Journal* (20 July 1855) 679–80.

44. See, for example, the report from the Select Committee on Protection of Infant Life, together with the proceedings of the Committee and Minutes of Evidence, 1871.

45. A. Bashford, *Purity and Pollution: Gender, Embodiment and Victorian Medicine* (London: Macmillan Press Ltd, 1998) pp. 63–83.

46. A. Nuttall, 'Passive Trust or Active Application: Changes in the Management of Difficult Childbirth and the Edinburgh Royal Maternity Hospital, 1850–1890', *Medical History*, 50 (2006) 351–72.

47. Other factors also contributed to closure: its much-admired leader, Mary Jones of St John's House, had problems with religious supervision; the villages most in need of midwives were unable to pledge the required income, while new applicants found six months' absence from home and the concomitant loss of earnings difficult to bear. See H. J. Betts, 'A Biographical Investigation of the Nightingale School for Midwives', Southampton University, Ed.D thesis (2002). See also Donnison, *Midwives*, p. 77.

48. Bashford, *Purity*, p. 67; J. H. Aveling, *English Midwives: Their History and Prospects* (London: J. & A. Churchill, 1872) p. 161, quoting the College prospectus.
49. F. Nightingale, *Introductory Notes on Lying-In Institutions, together with a Proposal for Organising an Institution for Training Midwives and Midwifery Nurses* (London: Longman, Green and Co., 1871) p. 106.
50. Nonetheless, it has been argued that the College made a major contribution to the rehabilitation of midwifery. See Donnison, *Midwives*, pp. 82–90.
51. Aveling, *English Midwives*, p. 158.
52. McIntosh, 'Profession', pp. 405–6.
53. Stephenson, 'Voluntary Maternity Hospital', pp. 197–8.
54. In November 1870, medical students in Matthews Duncan's extramural midwifery class complained at the presence of five females, including four nurses from the ERMH of 'inferior social status'. See *British Medical Journal* (12 November 1870) 541. At least one nurse owned a set of midwifery lecture notes made by a medical student. See EUL, DC10.36, DC10.35 1&2.
55. Nuttall, 'Edinburgh Royal Maternity Hospital', pp. 266–70.
56. *British Medical Journal* (29 August 1868) 227; (6 January 1872) 21.
57. McIntosh, 'Profession', Table 1, p. 409.
58. For example, in 1898 Anne Fraser of Killiecrankie was sent by the Duchess of Atholl; in 1897, 'Beatrice Callander, soldier's widow from Perth' attended, while the February 1896 class included six widows among 13 pupils; Anne G. Baillie (1899) 'had been a domestic servant'. See EUL, LHSA, ERMH, Register of Nurses 1892–1923, LHB3/20/1.
59. T. Ferguson, *Scottish Social Welfare* (Edinburgh: E. & S. Livingstone Ltd, 1958) p. 511. Matthews Duncan left Edinburgh for London in 1877.
60. Report from the Select Committee on Midwives' Registration, together with the Proceedings of the Committee and Minutes of Evidence, ordered by the House of Commons, Parliamentary Papers, 1892 (289) XIV, evidence of Dr A. D. L. Napier, p. 5.
61. Stephenson, 'Voluntary Maternity Hospital', pp. 26–39; L. Marks, 'Mothers, Babies and Hospitals: "The London" and the Provision of Maternity Care in East London, 1870–1939', in V. Fildes, L. Marks and H. Marland (eds), *Women and Children First: International Maternal and Infant Welfare 1870–1945* (London: Routledge, 1992) pp. 48–72.
62. Aveling, *English Midwives*, pp. 163–8.
63. Aveling, *English Midwives*, pp. 164–5.
64. Report from the Select Committee on Midwives' Registration, together with the Proceedings of the Committee and Minutes of Evidence (continued), Parliamentary Papers, 1893 (367) XIII, evidence of

Dr A. B. Hicks, pp. 22–4; Nuttall, 'Passive Trust', pp. 365–8. See also *Nursing Notes*, 11 (1898) 150 for the editorial comment following the use of ergot by a midwife, that 26 years ago it 'was not an uncommon practice with medical men, and, doubtless, [she] . . . was taught . . . to use ergot . . . under certain circumstances'.

65. Select Committee on Midwives' Registration, 1892, evidence of Dr W. M. G. Hewitt, p. 1149.
66. Aveling, *English Midwives*, p. 165.
67. *British Medical Journal* (24 February 1872) 224.
68. *Nursing Notes*, 4 (1891) 115, 99.
69. Donnison, *Midwives*, pp. 86–90.
70. Zepherina Veitch trained at University College Hospital in 1868, and was the tenth LOS diplomate. She later married the surgeon Professor Henry Smith.
71. Rosalind Paget was a niece of the philanthropist William Rathbone and of independent means.
72. They were supported by the Women's Liberal Federation, the doctor-led Midwives' Registration Association and 'a lay association of ladies', the Association for Promoting the Training and Compulsory Registration of Midwives. See *Nursing Notes*, 8 (1895) 2.
73. From 1888, *Nursing Notes* was produced independently by its editor and proprietor, Emma Brierly, and published by the Women's Printing Society Ltd. Early losses were met by Misses Paget and Brierly. See Cowell and Wainwright, *Blue Door*, pp. 20–1.
74. Cowell and Wainwright, *Blue Door*, pp. 15–16.
75. *Nursing Notes*, 13 (1900) 146.
76. *Nursing Notes*, 11 (1898) 50, 36; 4 (1891) 50. See also Heagerty, 'Handmaidens', pp. 74–6.
77. For example, the 180 medical students who attended the ERMH in 1890 apparently obscured the number of deliveries they actually conducted. See Nuttall, 'Edinburgh Royal Maternity Hospital', pp. 282–4.
78. Cowell and Wainwright, *Blue Door*, p. 26. ERMH physicians were intimidated into withdrawing their midwives' lecture certificates. See LHSA, ERMH Medical Board Minutes, 11 January 1893, 16 July 1894 [LHB 3/2/1].
79. See, in particular, Select Committee on Midwives' Registration, 1892, evidence of Dr R. R. Rentoul, pp. 345–689; Donnison, *Midwives*, pp. 127–39, 148–9.
80. Select Committee on Midwives' Registration (continued), 1893–4, Report, p. 3.
81. Mrs. Layton, 'Memories of Seventy Years', in M. L. Davies (ed.), *Life as We Have Known It* (London: Virago, 1977) p. 45.
82. Cowell and Wainwright, *Blue Door*, pp. 34–5.

83. Heagerty, 'Class', pp. iii, 23–4; Donnison, *Midwives*, pp. 176–7; Cowell and Wainwright, *Blue Door*, p. 45.
84. Cowell and Wainwright, *Blue Door*, p. 42.
85. The People's Story, Edinburgh Museums and Galleries, H. L. Hewitt, CMB certificate (No. 13889) [HH 6345/10/2004], ERMH certificate [HH 6345/9/2004] and midwife's bag [HH6345/1/2004].
86. *Nursing Notes*, 16 (1904) 71.
87. *Nursing Notes*, 17 (1905) 2; 16 (1904) 155.
88. Heagerty, 'Class', p. 92; Heagerty, 'Handmaidens', pp. 78–82; Donnison, *Midwives*, p. 180.
89. Dale and Fisher, 'Implementing the 1902 Midwives Act', 446–8, 439, 443.
90. Mottram, 'State Control', pp. 141–6.
91. McIntosh, 'Profession', p. 419.
92. I. Jones, 'Elizabeth Davies, Midwife, 1853–1927', *The London Hospital Gazette*, 73 (1970) 9–12.
93. F. Nic Suibhne, 'On the Straw' and Other Aspects of Pregnancy and Childbirth from the Oral Tradition of Women in Ulster', *Ulster Folklife*, 38 (1992) 12–24.
94. Donnison, *Midwives*, pp. 154–6.
95. *Nursing Notes*, 16 (1904) 99.
96. *Nursing Notes*, 16 (1904) 115.
97. *The Midwives Record* (May 1910) 138, cited in Heagerty, 'Class', pp. 106–11; Heagerty, 'Handmaidens', pp. 82–7.
98. Nuttall, 'Edinburgh Royal Maternity Hospital', pp. 312–3.
99. See F. Thompson, *Lark Rise to Candleford* (Harmondsworth: Penguin Modern Classics, 1980) pp. 135–6 for descriptions of kindly Mrs Quinton, who saw 'the beginning and end of everybody', and her supercilious certified replacement. See also *Maternity: Letters from Working-Women*, Women's Co-operative Guild (New York: Garland Publishing, 1980) pp. 124–8 for an account of a 'know-it-all' certified midwife who doubted her patient's knowledge of her own body. Bergin reports a similar attitude to Jubilee nurse-midwives in Ireland. (Bergin, 'Childbirth').
100. Donnison, *Midwives*, p. 182.
101. Reid, *Midwifery in Scotland*, pp. 30–7, 40–1, 47–8.
102. 'Editorial', *Lancet* (18 June 1910) 1699, cited in McMahon, 'Regulating Midwives', p. 167.
103. McMahon, 'Regulating Midwives', p. 171.

7

Midwifery, 1920–2000: The Reshaping of a Profession

Billie Hunter

The twentieth century was a period of transformation for British midwives, with midwives' role and status undergoing significant changes. However, this transformation was not always smooth or straightforward. As the following account suggests, the period was characterized by new clinical developments and contrasting approaches to maternity care, which in turn influenced the role of the midwife. At times, these changes stimulated an energetic response from the profession, while at other times there was a notable silence.

> When I saw the modern labour room it was very different from what I had been used to [...] She pointed out this machine and that [...]. My eyes were like organ stops and I said, 'I don't know how to work the bed pan machine let alone all this [...] however, put me on top of Ben Lidi with somebody having twins and I would be able to cope'.[1]

Key changes during the period relate to training, employment, scope of practice and locus of care. In 1920, midwives commonly worked in self-employed independent practice, having undertaken apprenticeship-style training in a hospital-based midwifery school. Most births took place at home, with the midwife taking full responsibility for uncomplicated pregnancies. The emphasis was on the normalcy of childbirth, and normal childbirth was seen as the midwife's territory.[2] In contrast, by the end of the twentieth century increasing numbers of midwives were graduates, working mainly within the National Health Service (NHS) in either hospital or community. Most births took place in hospital, with technological surveillance of pregnancy and birth seen as routine. Despite significant improvements in maternal and infant mortality since the 1920s, birth was increasingly seen as normal 'only in retrospect',[3] a risky process requiring scientific control and management by obstetricians. This chapter analyses these changes, setting the evolution of midwifery in its broader social and political context. The histories of both midwifery and maternity care are considered as interwoven threads in the same tapestry, with shifts in the conceptualization of childbirth inevitably affecting the work of the midwife. In particular, the chapter considers how the pursuit of professionalization and shifting political debates related to place of birth and professional territories have influenced the midwife's role.

Three key periods will be discussed, in which the most significant developments occurred: 1920–37, which saw early professionalization and the move to a salaried service; 1938–74, when the effects of the Second World War and the NHS were experienced; and post-1974, when battle was waged between the competing paradigms of technology and nature.

The New Professional Midwife, 1920–37

Much of the latter part of the nineteenth century was taken up in campaigning for state regulation of midwifery, culminating in the 1902 Midwives' Act in England and Wales, and the Midwives (Scotland) Act in 1915.[4] Once this legislation was in place, the task for midwifery leaders was to establish midwifery as a respectable profession, disassociated from untrained midwives or 'handywomen'. A series of Midwifery Acts followed (1918, 1926, 1936 in England and Wales; 1922, 1927, 1937 in Scotland), all of which increasingly restricted the role of the handywoman. Handywomen were still present at births, however, at least in a support role, until the 1940s.[5] It is unclear how much 'truth' there was in the many accusations of dangerous practice made against handywomen by midwifery leaders. *Nursing Notes*, the midwifery journal of the time, contains articles and letters which paint a vivid picture of the tensions that existed. For example, a letter concerning the Third Midwives Act (1926) notes that 'although the [Act] is not as strong as we wished, there is evidence that it can be an efficient weapon against the depredations of our foe "the handy lady" '.[6] In contrast, oral accounts suggest that many handywomen were valued and respected within their communities, providing kind, competent care and often working alongside trained midwives.[7]

There were high hopes for what midwives could achieve, particularly in relation to reducing maternal and infant mortality and improving public health. This was not only in relation to care during labour and childbirth. Interest was growing in the new concept of antenatal care, and its contribution to improving the health of the nation.[8] There was mounting concern about high levels of infant and maternal mortality, and pressure on the government to tackle these. In 1918, the Maternal and Child Welfare Act had required local authorities to establish maternal and child welfare centres, to include antenatal clinics.[9] It was envisaged that midwives would play a key role in this initiative, thus extending the scope of their practice.[10]

However, innovations in antenatal care were set against a backdrop of growing economic depression and social deprivation, which made the achievement of such goals unrealistic. High levels of unemployment, low household incomes, poor quality housing and inadequate diet led to widespread social unrest. The health and well-being of many mothers and babies was thus already compromised, and there was little that the ordinary midwife could do to alleviate such a heavy burden of disadvantage. As Elsie, a midwife who worked in Derby in the 1930s described to Leap and Hunter:

> The conditions were very bad. Filthy some of the back streets. They've all been demolished now. Very bad. If there was time, we used to wipe over the tops of the furniture before we laid our things out, but sometimes there was only just time to catch the baby and that was all.[11]

The contribution of midwives to public health was also compromised by the national shortage of midwives and difficult working conditions. Prior to the Second World War, most midwives practised in the community, although it was also possible to find employment in small maternity homes, as well as in the maternity departments of voluntary hospitals and Poor Law Infirmaries. It is estimated that during the 1930s between 60 per cent and 70 per cent of births occurred at home,[12] attended mainly by midwives working in independent practice. While these self-employed midwives had significant occupational autonomy, they also experienced many difficulties. The important 1917 report *The Physical Welfare of Mothers and Children*[13] had identified how the potentially valuable role of midwives in preventing infant and maternal mortality was often hampered by their working conditions. The author, Dr Janet Campbell, Senior Medical Officer in the Department of Maternal and Child Welfare at the Ministry of Health, drew attention to the demanding nature of self-employed, single-handed practice, highlighting midwives' high level of responsibility, poor remuneration, long hours and relative low status:[14] a picture supported by oral history evidence.[15]

The 1917 report had also raised concerns regarding the limited duration, financing and content of midwifery training. In response, in 1926 training was increased from six to twelve months for direct entrants, and from four to six months for nurse entrants.[16] Limited financial support became available. Previously, all training costs were covered by pupil midwives themselves, which inevitably prevented many working-class women from applying. From 1919, the Treasury made a small contribution of £20, on condition that the midwife guaranteed to practise on qualification.[17] Even so, this contribution barely covered living expenses.[18] Content of training was also questioned, as many 'pupil' midwives gained only community experience. A month-long period of hospital practice was recommended,[19] to include more attention to medical complications, suggesting that a trend towards institution-based birth was beginning.

Since the First World War, there had been growing pressure to increase institution-based maternity care, both in maternity homes and hospitals. This pressure came from a range of interested parties, each with different concerns. In the main, their focus was on responding to women's social needs rather than increasing clinical safety.[20] For example, user groups such as the Women's Co-operative Guild emphasized the need for working-class women to get sufficient rest during the lying-in period, which was often not achievable in their own homes. Obstetricians did emphasize clinical safety, although this was directed at women with complications.[21] For the time being at least, the attitude of the medical profession was that childbirth was a normal process. In the view of the British Medical Association, 'all the available evidence demonstrates that normal confinements, and those which show only a minor departure from normal, can be conducted more safely at home than in hospital'.[22]

Concerns regarding midwives' well-being and financial security continued, with Dr Janet Campbell championing their cause. In her follow-on report *The Training of Midwives* (1926), she argued that midwives needed to be educated to a high degree of competency if the prevailing high levels of maternal mortality were to be successfully tackled.[23] Her vision for improved midwifery status underpinned a campaign, led by the Birthday Trust, which eventually resulted in the 1936 Midwives' Act.[24] This Act required local councils to provide a salaried domiciliary midwifery service, subsidised by the government. Self-employed midwives were able to apply for salaried posts or continue in independent practice. In reality, few took the latter option.[25] Oral evidence suggests that there was great competition for these highly desirable salaried posts: '... it helped the local authority to weed out the ones they didn't want. It gave them more control over us. Some midwives didn't get jobs and it caused a lot of hard feeling.'[26]

The 1936 Midwives' Act has been said to have 'revolutionised the position and standard of practice of midwives'.[27] Midwives no longer had to ask for direct payment from their clients (who were expected instead to make a contribution to the local authority). Again, oral accounts suggest that this was a relief for many midwives, not only because it was an unpleasant task to ask for payment from families who were already living on the breadline, but also because it guaranteed financial security: 'before 1936, your income was very precarious, because you had what you earned [...] I've always been paid, but sometimes by instalments because people hadn't a lot of money in the early 1930s'.[28] There were other concurrent benefits for midwives' quality of life: midwives now had off-duty time, annual leave, and uniforms and equipment provided.

The Act also aimed to improve midwifery education: a Midwife Teacher's Diploma was introduced, and regular updating for qualified midwives began, in the form of compulsory seven-day refresher courses every five years. The recommendation that training be increased to two years for direct entrants and one year for nurses, with the course divided into equal lengths of community and hospital experience, was implemented in 1938.[29]

However, while the creation of a salaried service considerably improved the working conditions of midwives, it could also be argued that this came at a price. Midwives were now under greater state control and the parameters of practice were increasingly monitored by doctors and midwifery supervisors, with inevitable restrictions on occupational autonomy.

Although the goal of removing midwifery from what was perceived as the contaminating influence of the handywomen had been largely achieved, and the project of re-shaping midwifery as a profession was clearly underway, the extent to which the ambitious aims of the early reformers had been realized is questionable. There were many (growing) restrictions on midwives' scope of practice and autonomy. The medical profession maintained considerable involvement in both midwifery education and professional regulation, thus influencing the nature and scope of midwives' practice. It is likely that there was an economic basis to these restrictions. In the community particularly, midwives and family doctors were in direct competition for maternity 'patients' and, prior to the formation of the NHS, this meant that economic livelihoods were at stake. Rivalry for custom was somewhat ameliorated by the introduction of a salaried midwifery service, but this brought with it both benefits and limitations. Independent midwifery practice became increasingly rare, and did not become a significant element of midwifery again until its renaissance in the 1970s.

The Effects of the Second World War and the Formation of the NHS, 1948–74

However, all these concerns were overtaken by the Second World War. Emergency Medical Services (EMS) were set up, and maternity care was treated as high priority.[30] The birth rate was high throughout the 1940s, reaching a peak in 1946. As there was a shortage of midwives, midwifery was designated as a form of national service in order to encourage retired and non-working midwives to return to practice.[31] Midwifery-run maternity homes were set up in rural areas, often in requisitioned country houses far away from cities under threat of bombing, and many pregnant women from the cities were evacuated.[32]

Despite the challenges of wartime work, midwives described enjoying many aspects of their work in this period, particularly their increased autonomy and the sense of female camaraderie.[33] There were also improvements in the health and well-being of women and their babies. The maternal mortality rate began to fall dramatically after the mid-1930s,[34] reaching 2.3 per 1,000 births in 1943, half of the 1935 rate.[35] This was partly attributable to improvements in clinical care, such as the introduction of antibiotics and blood transfusion services. The wartime fortified rations and supplements provided to pregnant and nursing mothers are also likely to have been significant.

The contribution of midwives to the war effort was acknowledged in the 1943 Rushcliffe Report.[36] This report is particularly interesting as it makes a clear distinction between the nursing and midwifery professions, noting the increased autonomy and responsibility of midwives and recommending that this be reflected in slightly higher salary scales. However, the Report's underlying motives have been questioned. Dingwall et al. suggest, for example, that the emphasis on midwives' independence was a retention strategy designed mainly to 'keep midwives at work by persuasion, flattery and cajolery'.[37]

The EMS strategies, in particular the recommendation for institution-based birth, influenced the post-war changes to maternity services which occurred as part of NHS formation. The NHS offered universal health care free at the point of delivery, including the provision of maternity care. While this offered many potential benefits for the health of women and babies, the formation of the NHS had major implications for midwifery: hospital birth rates increased dramatically, thus shifting the main locus of care, and general practitioners (GPs) became the first point of contact for pregnant women. These changes are considered in turn.

The continued increase in hospital birth rates during and following the war does not appear to have been merely a pragmatic response to social needs.[38] A fundamental shift in medical and social attitudes towards childbirth was also evident. In 1944, a report by the Royal College of Obstetricians and Gynaecologists had recommended that maternity hospital accommodation should be expanded so that 70 per cent of births could be provided for;[39] ten years later they were recommending 100 per cent provision.[40] The shift in attitudes to childbirth is also evident in the titles of these documents: the 1944 document reports on the 'national *maternity service*', whereas the 1954 Report focuses on 'the *obstetric service* under the NHS'.

Public demand for hospital births increased, later supported by campaigning groups such as the Association for Improvements in Maternity Services (AIMS) when this was formed in 1960.[41] Several reasons for this have been suggested. There was increased public belief in the ability of medical science to improve outcomes. Attitudes towards hospital care were also changing, as NHS hospitals became emblematic of 'the bright new world of medical science triumphant',[42] replacing negative memories of workhouses and Poor Law Infirmaries. The prospect of free hospital care and rest may also have proved an attractive alternative to the disruption and expense created by a home birth, especially for working-class women.[43] Many women were also increasingly requesting analgesia during childbirth. Although community midwives (known at the time as domiciliary or district midwives) were able to give some pain relief at home, stronger analgesia could only be provided within a hospital.[44]

The increase in hospital births meant that the ratio of hospital- and community-based midwives needed to change and roles needed to become more demarcated. Community midwives were much less likely to attend births, and their work became more focused on antenatal and postnatal care. In contrast, hospital midwives provided all aspects of care, but within an environment that was increasingly focused on the surveillance and management of childbirth.

The introduction of the NHS also altered the respective roles of community midwife and GP. Maternity care was now accessed via the GP, who received payment for providing his/her services.[45] The GP would refer the woman to the midwife, rather than the previous practice where women booked with the midwife, who referred to the GP as necessary. This fundamentally altered the power dynamic in this relationship, as the midwife no longer competed with the GP for clients, but had become his subordinate.[46] A midwife who worked 'on the district' from 1931 to 1968 clearly attributed the erosion of the midwife's role to the introduction of the NHS:

> The midwife's status has gone down such a lot recently. It started at around the time of the NHS Act, I think, when the doctors started doing more and more antenatal care and the midwives said, 'Oh well, the doctor gets paid for it – he'll do it'. Instead of sticking up for their own status, they let their status go, and that's where the midwives started to go down.[47]

The 1949 Central Midwives Board (CMB) Annual Report expressed concerns about the decreasing number of home births and the increased role of the GP in normal midwifery, cautioning that this would affect the education and practice of future midwives. The Board proposed that home birth should remain the norm, with hospitalization only for high-risk cases.[48]

However, the trend was set to continue. The selection criteria for hospitalized birth were being widened and the number of consultant beds increased from the late 1950s onwards. The emphasis shifted from identifying high-risk women who would benefit from consultant care to selecting those who were considered sufficiently low risk to be 'allowed' a home delivery. The underpinning assumption was that mortality rates would be decreased by hospital delivery, although it is now generally acknowledged that this assumption was untested and based on spurious explanations of causality.[49] It is important to note, however, that obstetricians had the support of consumer groups in this initiative. Pressure groups such as the National Childbirth Trust were campaigning for the right to a hospital bed and effective analgesia for all.[50]

The NHS changes created a complicated system of maternity care. The Guillebaud Report, charged with investigating the costs of the NHS, had identified that the maternity services were in 'a state of some confusion, which must impair their usefulness and which should not be allowed to continue'.[51] In response, in 1956 the Cranbrook Committee commenced a review of maternity services in England and Wales.[52] Many concerns were identified: service organization was complicated, with hospital and community midwives being managed separately; care was fragmented and lacked co-ordination, so that women and their babies would be seen by numerous professionals and care would often be duplicated. However, rather than recommending the creation of a new amalgamated service, the proposed solution was to increase the numbers of hospital births to 70 per cent. This was seen as a more viable option than reorganization, as it was argued that this would necessitate restructuring the entire NHS.[53]

The National Birthday Trust Fund, an influential charity which had campaigned since the 1920s to improve maternity care and decrease maternal and infant mortality rates, expressed concern about the proposals. Giving evidence to the Cranbrook Committee, its leaders argued that the projected additional 200,000 hospital births would require new maternity hospitals to be built and staffed. As there was already a shortage of midwives, this was clearly problematic. Retention of midwives was difficult: of 5,000 pupils taking Part One of the CMB examination, only an estimated 800 were practising as midwives three years later. The Trust also cautioned that the proposals would lead to the decline of community-based maternity care, which they considered essential for optimizing public health and reducing mortality. Instead, the Trustees recommended a unified hospital and district maternity service, with additional support for midwives being provided by semi-skilled maternity nurses and nursing assistants 'of a type who would not be capable of passing examinations of the same difficulty as those of fully qualified professional midwives. [...] A percentage of candidates might be coloured women, many of whom might well prove to be of great value.'[54] At the time of the the Cranbrook Review, the Ministry of Health and Labour was actively campaigning to recruit health-care staff from the Colonies, in order to address workforce shortages in the United Kingdom. The suggestion that 'coloured women' would be best suited to semiskilled maternity work was congruent with the dominant thinking of that time, where it was argued that intellectual capacity and career motivation were limited by 'racial characteristics'.[55] For women arriving from the Caribbean in search of enhanced professional career opportunities, this semi-skilled role may have been far from what they imagined, and there is evidence that many women were duped into training for roles that offered little in the way of future career progression.[56]

The Royal College of Midwives (RCM) also expressed concerns about midwifery retention, cautioning in a memorandum to the Cranbrook Committee that there was 'a grave shortage of midwives in some maternity hospitals and homes [....] The need is not so much to attract more recruits into midwifery training as to retain the trained personnel in the practice of midwifery.'[57] The memorandum, however, mainly focused on negotiating the future role of the midwife in relation to doctors, implying an acceptance of increased medical involvement in maternity care. Midwives were now characterized as members of the 'obstetric team' working 'in association with doctors'.[58]

Despite RCM recommendations that 'although a doctor may be present for part of the time, the midwife should take full responsibility for the majority of normal deliveries',[59] the eventual Cranbrook Report recommended an increased role for doctors: 'a general practitioner obstetrician should, wherever possible, attend all domiciliary confinements, to safeguard the mother and baby against unforeseen emergencies.... The conduct of a normal confinement is the *joint responsibility* of the doctor and midwife' (my italics).[60] This represented a major shift in professional roles and responsibilities. The assumed additional expertise and seniority of the GP implicit in the Report led to an expectation that midwives would defer to medical opinion and act as medical assistants, even in uncomplicated cases.[61] Although the Cranbrook Report went on to state that 'nothing should be done to lessen the importance of the midwife',[62] this would appear to be nothing more than a token gesture to appease the RCM, given that the Report was clearly advocating a diminished midwifery role.

During the 1960s, the consequences of these changes for both community and hospital midwives became increasingly apparent. Community midwives were much less likely to attend births, and indeed the bulk of their time was taken up in providing postnatal care, often to women whom they did not know. This was partially the result of Early Discharge Schemes, introduced in the early 1960s as the solution to the shortage of hospital beds resulting from increased hospital births.[63] Early discharge increased the community midwives' workload, both in the postnatal period, and also antenatally, as the midwife was required to assess the 'appropriateness' of home conditions.

The work of hospital midwives changed with the introduction of centralized 'delivery suites'. Before the 1960s, women had usually received all their hospital care, including support during labour and birth, on the same ward.[64] The introduction of new large delivery suites resulted in a service more akin to a conveyor belt, with women passing through the various departments of the unit for different aspects of their care.[65] Care was thus fragmented, as was the midwife's role. Midwives increasingly specialized in differing aspects of maternity care, and risked losing the full range of their expertise. The introduction of new technologies such as the 'Cardiff pump' for induction of labour required hospital midwives to acquire new technical skills, compounding their position as obstetric nurses, rather than 'practitioners in their own right'.[66] The expertise of the midwife in normal birth began to seem old-fashioned and outdated.

Surprisingly, given the implications of these developments, there appears to have been little resistance either from individual midwives or from those representing the profession until the 1970s. The CMB was supportive of the Cranbrook Report's recommendations, stating that in their opinion the 'main purposes of the 1902 Midwives Act have been fulfilled'.[67] Given their concern two years earlier regarding the effects of increased hospitalization of birth on the role of the community midwife, their positive response to the Report is surprising and suggests a lack of long-term vision. Tew observes that 'there is no record for over thirty years of any effective opposition by organised midwives to the relentless rejection of their philosophy and the erosion of their traditional service'.[68] This lack of resistance could have many causes, although this is difficult to ascertain as research evidence is limited for this period. It may be that midwives were convinced by the claims that increased medical and technological involvement would improve maternity care. Individual dissenters may have felt silenced by the majority view, as well as by the authoritative voice of obstetric medicine. It is highly likely that gender and professional status influenced 'whose knowledge counted'[69] in this period. Midwifery certainly lacked a unified voice, largely the result of the growing divisions between hospital-based and community-based midwifery. Whatever the cause, it was not until the 1970s that any concerted opposition began, led by maternity service users.

Post-1974: Competing Paradigms

The period from 1974 to 2000 was a time of rapid change for midwifery, characterized by tensions resulting from conflicting approaches to childbirth and their implications for the midwife's role. Growing professional and lay interest in 'natural' childbirth prompted a radical grass-roots challenge to medical intervention which later influenced government policy. There was also another significant attempt to increase the professional status of midwives, this time via a shift in approaches to education: 'training courses' became 'educational programmes', eventually provided within universities. There were growing aspirations to base practice on research evidence, and midwives began to make their own contribution to the body of maternity-related research.

During the 1970s, hospital birth was almost universal. The 1970 Peel Report recommended that 'the resources of modern medicine should be available to all mothers and babies, and we think that sufficient facilities should be provided to allow for 100% hospital delivery'.[70] Obstetric technologies were being rapidly developed, so that interventions such as induction of labour, electronic monitoring and epidural analgesia became almost routine, even in low-risk cases.[71] These innovations also established obstetrics as an interesting branch of medical science, raising its status within medical specialisms. The opportunities offered by ultrasonic scans for surveillance of the growing foetus and innovations in assisted conception (such as in vitro fertilization) further added to its appeal.

Increased obstetric intervention had a major impact on public and professional perceptions of childbirth. Definitions of normality and abnormality were being re-constructed. Rather than pregnancy and labour being considered normal until proved otherwise, all childbirth was now viewed as potentially risky, to be classified as normal 'only in retrospect'.[72] This significant shift in approach placed pregnancy and birth firmly in the medical domain, so that the traditional view of midwives as the experts in normal childbirth was no longer credible. As Kirkham argues, in effect midwives were 'defined out of existence'.[73] The reality for many midwives was that they were re-created as maternity nurses with minimal autonomy.[74] Although midwives still had more discretion in their practice than nurses, they were ultimately constrained by 'a framework of rules defined by modern obstetric practice'.[75]

Medicalization also undermined the traditional knowledge of midwives, characterized by 'masterful inactivity' and one-to-one support, replacing it with a 'scientific' approach characterized by use of technology and 'active management' of labour.[76] At this time, midwives had little evidence to support the value of their traditional 'low-tech' approach to childbirth, and the technological culture swiftly became accepted as 'authoritative knowledge'.[77] The 'legitimacy and authority of midwifery' had been fundamentally challenged.[78]

Community midwives had more opportunities than their hospital counterparts to retain some degree of autonomy. However, this was compromised to some extent by the National Health Service Reorganisation Act of 1973. This created the long-awaited unification of maternity services, with 'Nursing' Officers responsible for managing both hospital and community midwives. Towler and Bramall, from their firsthand experience of this period, claim that this change was 'psychologically traumatic to some community midwives and also to some managers',[79] as fundamental differences in the needs of hospital and community staff were apparently ignored. Community midwives became attached to GP practices, rather than local authority clinics. While this may have increased the opportunities for teamworking, it also gave GPs further power to determine the extent of midwifery involvement during pregnancy.

Challenges to Medicalization

In the same period, a user-led challenge to routine medicalization of childbirth was gathering momentum, grounded in other contemporary movements for social change such as feminism, consumer health movements and 'natural' alternatives to bio-medicine. A number of articulate childbirth campaigners, including the anthropologist Sheila Kitzinger and the French obstetrician Michel Odent, led the challenge, in collaboration with service user organizations such as the National Childbirth Trust (which had now shifted its position to promoting women's choice in place of birth), the Maternity Alliance, the Active Birth Movement and the Association for Improvements in Maternity Services (AIMS). The initiative was predominantly user-led, with some professional participation evident. There was a proliferation in literature which questioned the extent of clinical intervention in childbirth and the need for hospitalized birth.[80]

In particular, unnecessary interventions such as routine inductions and episiotomies were rigorously questioned.[81]

In these campaigns, the role of the midwife was considered integral to improving maternity care and 'humanising' childbirth. Midwifery became something of a feminist cause, as Sheila Kitzinger explained:

> the new midwifery has a vital part to play in the women's movement... [it] gives vivid expression to the way in which women are discovering strength and sisterhood as we turn to help and support one another during the intense, exhilarating and powerful experience of childbirth.[82]

Midwifery was reclaimed as a valuable career for women and feminist women chose to enter midwifery as a means of expressing their feminism.[83] Once again midwifery was being re-shaped. The key protagonists were the members of the Association of Radical Midwives (ARM). Formed in 1976 as a support and study group, its members shared concerns regarding the erosion of the midwife's role and what was perceived as the resulting poor quality care for women. The Association quickly evolved into a political action group, whose position was clearly situated in feminism.[84] Gender issues were central to the analysis of the state of maternity care: midwives and women were seen as being similarly disempowered by medicalization, so that an alliance between midwives and mothers, based on their common experiences as women, was constructed as the way forward. Midwives were urged to reclaim their traditional skills and 'with woman' role. From early on, continuity of care was envisaged as the means by which both women and midwives could redress the balance of power.[85] In essence, ARM was arguing for a return to midwifery as it had been practised before the 1936 Act. This analysis remains evident in midwifery literature today.

Whether the views of ARM members were representative of British midwives in general is debatable. A survey of midwives' opinions revealed that only 14 per cent agreed with ARM's central claim that midwives had become little more than obstetric nurses. Most were happy with their role, confident in their level of skill and dismissive of the idea that fragmented care led to de-skilling.[86] Weitz suggests that this difference can be explained by the higher educational status of ARM members and their identification with feminism. For these midwives, the overt ideology of ARM provided 'an intellectual framework [. . .] to analyze their work experiences in political terms and to define their position as oppressive rather than simply unfortunate'.[87]

Although its membership was relatively small, the significance of ARM should not be underestimated in any analysis of the profession's recent history. It provided a discourse for midwifery that filled the existing void, and a strategic approach to influencing the political and professional agenda. Many of its members became active in a variety of 'official' fields, such as education, research and management. The publication of *The Vision*[88] in 1986 enabled ARM to demonstrate that its objectives were rational, carefully considered and supported by research evidence. *The Vision's* objectives included increased midwife autonomy via community-based group practices, with midwives providing continuity of care for the majority of women. ARM kept its finger on the political pulse, responding to government documents and providing an alternative response to that of the RCM.

The 'radicalization' of midwifery in the 1970s and 1980s was also evident in the re-emergence of independent midwifery, advocated as a means of increasing autonomy and job satisfaction. This was the first time since the 1936 Act that midwives were opting to work in independent practice. While numbers of independent midwives have remained small, and have faced many challenges, they have continued to play a significant role as alternative role models.

Alongside these radical initiatives, however, other changes were taking place that were less conducive to increasing the professional status of midwifery. The CMB was abolished in 1979, to be superseded by the United Kingdom Central Council for Nursing, Midwifery and Health Visiting (UKCC) and four National Boards. For the first time in 77 years, there was no separate regulatory body for midwives (although a specific Midwifery Committee was established within the UKCC), which led to fears that midwifery would be subsumed by nursing. NHS reorganization meant that many midwives were now managed by nurses, leading to concerns that the midwifery perspective would not be effectively represented. These concerns were further exacerbated by the Project 2000 proposals for nurse training,[89] which recommended that midwifery become a specialist branch of nursing. This proposal had its roots in the 1972 Briggs Report, which recommended that all future midwives should be nurses.[90] These proposals were fiercely rejected by midwives and led to a brief (unsuccessful) campaign for a new Midwives' Act.[91]

The Renaissance of Midwifery?

Perhaps galvanized by this challenge, midwifery was about to undergo something of a renaissance. The distinctiveness of midwifery from nursing was emphasized in publications and policies. Direct-entry midwifery education was suddenly back in fashion, after a steady decline, which had meant that, at its lowest ebb in 1983, it was offered by only one midwifery school. ARM had identified direct entry as the means by which midwifery could be re-established as a profession with a distinct identity.[92] Direct entrant students were considered better able to resist the dominance of the bio-medical model and to be more likely to see themselves as doctors' equals, unlike students already trained as nurses who, it was argued, would already have been socialized into the dominant value system of the NHS. The idea was taken up by the Department of Health, and by 1989 the government paper *Working for Patients*[93] recommended expansion of direct-entry midwifery. Between 1989 and 1993, 35 new direct-entry programmes were established in England. The reasons given for this 'U-turn', however, were pragmatic rather than ideological: as, unlike nurse-trained midwives, direct entrants could practice only as midwives, it was a cost-effective strategy for ensuring retention of the midwifery workforce.

The radical principles of ARM were clearly visible in the far-reaching changes to maternity care proposed in the 1990s. The 1992 *Winterton Report*[94] argued that there was no evidence to support 100 per cent hospitalization for birth and recommended that a medical model of care should no longer dominate. In response to this controversial report, an Expert Maternity Group chaired by Baroness Cumberlege was charged with reviewing maternity policy and making specific recommendations about future maternity services in England. A widespread consultation exercise was undertaken, gathering information from a range of professionals and users of the service.

The recommendations of the Group's report, *Changing Childbirth,* were extensive. In brief, its key principles were that women and their families should receive individualized care and be fully involved in decision-making; that maternity services should be primarily community-based, accessible and responsive to local needs; and that care should be effective and efficient.[95] Midwives were to play a full role in maternity care, using all their skills and knowledge. Women with uncomplicated pregnancies could choose a midwife as their main care provider and choose where to give birth, thus raising the possibility of an increased home birth rate. It should be noted that *Changing Childbirth* was an English report, and other UK countries had their own policies, for example, the Welsh Office *Protocol for Investment in Health Gain: Maternal and Early Child Health.*[96] However, *Changing Childbirth* was discussed throughout the United Kingdom and its recommendations were clearly influential in the maternity and midwifery policies of all UK countries.

A number of factors appear to have prompted these radical recommendations. Firstly, the cost–effectiveness of centralized maternity care was being questioned, as there was little evidence to support this in terms of safety for mother and baby.[97] Secondly, there was increasing empirical evidence that medicalized childbirth was not only expensive but often of no proven benefit or even potentially harmful.[98] This critique was informed by a 'totally new culture'[99] within the NHS: an emphasis on 'evidence-based practice', where effectiveness had been demonstrated by research. Thirdly, service user criticism of maternity care was well documented and increasingly hard to ignore, especially as, Sandall[100] observes, the Conservative government of the time espoused the principle of consumer choice.

The practical implications of the report were profound. The recommendation that midwives should work flexibly across community and hospital settings in order to provide continuity of care fundamentally altered both the context and content of midwives' work. However, the report did not specify how continuity of care should be organized, recommending that units devise their own 'models and strategies'.[101] This lack of prescriptiveness could be perceived as enabling and liberating for midwifery; alternatively, it could be argued that the lack of guidance (and funding) to implement the changes would ultimately result in failure.

Midwives were divided in their reactions, as apparent in the midwifery press of the time. Many were enthusiastic, seeing this as the opportunity to resurrect midwifery.[102] Others raised doubts regarding the feasibility of the proposals,[103] questioning the achievability of continuity of care and its practical implications for midwives' working lives. Not surprisingly, the report received a lukewarm reception from obstetricians and GPs. The report was eventually published as a consultation document, rather than as policy as originally intended. By 2000, many *Changing Childbirth* projects had ceased to exist, although its principles remain evident in many subsequent UK policies.[104]

One particular criticism of *Changing Childbirth* was its lack of attention to social inequalities and their impact on maternity outcomes.[105] These issues came to the forefront as the century came to a close, when once again the public health role of the midwife was acknowledged. Although some public health concerns were new (e.g. the health needs of the increased black and ethnic minority population), other concerns were more longstanding and resistant to improvement (e.g. the impact of social class and income on perinatal mortality rates).

A New Professional Project?

At the same time as *Changing Childbirth* was recommending that midwives reclaim their professional role as experts in normal childbirth, there were concurrent initiatives to enhance the professional status of midwives. Academic qualifications, research and scholarship were identified as the modern route to professionalization. In the late 1980s and early 1990s, midwifery education moved into universities, and the first degree courses began. There was increasing emphasis on midwifery's distinctiveness from nursing, and direct-entry midwifery programmes continued to flourish. Approaches to education changed: university curricula were required to be evidence-based, and aimed at developing the critical thinking skills of practitioners, a far cry from the rote learning that epitomized the training of midwives earlier in the century.

Midwives were far from united in their response to this move, however, with many questioning whether it would create a gulf between theory and practice and reduce clinical skills.[106] The move into higher education certainly presented (and continues to present) many challenges, as many midwifery educationalists lacked a natural 'fit' within academia, frequently missing the usual academic credentials of a doctoral qualification and research track record. They also were often distanced, both physically and ideologically, from clinical colleagues, who expressed concerns that the 'hands-on' and vocational aspects of midwifery could be lost if midwifery lecturers relinquished their links with practice to meet academic demands.

Despite these reservations, midwifery made rapid progress in developing its academic profile and used this to enhance its professional status. By developing the scientific basis for their practice, midwives aimed to produce quantitative and qualitative evidence which would both support a 'midwifery', as opposed to obstetric, approach to maternity care and also demonstrate its value. Beginning in the 1980s, a number of influential midwife-led studies were published, which challenged existing practice.[107] These studies formed part of the new NHS 'evidence-based practice' culture, in which maternity care research, led by Iain Chalmers and the National Perinatal Epidemiology Unit at Oxford University, was playing a key role. Evidence-based practice appeared to provide midwives with the opportunity, and the rationale, to challenge the wisdom of previous interventionist approaches to maternity care.

Conclusion

Between 1920 and 2000 midwifery experienced many changes. There have been periods of great activity and development, and other periods of apparent resigned acceptance. Although it could be argued that midwifery was in a much stronger position at the end of the century than in the 1920s, with a clearer identity and stronger claim to professional status, on closer inspection it can be seen that many areas of ambiguity and tension remained.

A number of common themes are apparent in the analysis offered by this chapter. Midwifery is a small gendered occupation, provided largely by women for women. It is thus in danger of being marginalized, seen as 'women's business' which lacks relevance to wider health-care concerns. Midwifery services are difficult to manage and forward planning is tricky, as birth rates are erratic and childbirth itself is unpredictable. Midwifery has been dogged by frequent workforce shortages, largely due to problems with retention rather than recruitment. A number of solutions have been attempted, including improving pay and conditions and introducing a variety of support worker roles. The obduracy of the problem suggests that there are deeper-seated causes which need closer investigation.

Midwifery has also suffered from its lack of distinctiveness from nursing. This was particularly acute during the 1980s, when direct-entry programmes were all but extinct and midwifery looked likely to be subsumed into nursing. While midwives hold dear the concept of being an autonomous practitioner in their own right, and use this to differentiate their role from that of nurses, in reality restricted autonomy has been problematic for midwives since the formation of the NHS. The differing roles of midwives and doctors also became increasingly unclear after 1948, with blurred territories and competing claims for occupational jurisdiction. These ambiguities have all been influenced by changing and conflicting approaches to childbirth, in particular whether it is conceptualized as a normal or risky process. There is little evidence of a united midwifery voice over these 80 years. A lack of consensus about the way forward is characteristic, particularly in relation to achieving professionalization. A variety of professional projects have been attempted, the most recent proposing to accomplish professional status via academia and research. It is unclear, however, whether these various professional projects have always been congruent with the everyday concerns of 'grass-roots' midwives. If they merely reflect the ambitions of a minority, then their limited success is hardly surprising.

Notes

1. L. Reid, *Scottish Midwives: Twentieth Century Voices* (Dunfermline: Black Devon Books, 2008), interview with Ella Clelland, p. 125
2. N. Leap and B. Hunter, *The Midwife's Tale* (London: Scarlet Press, 1993).
3. R. Percival, 'Management of Normal Labour', *The Practitioner*, 1221 (1970) 204.
4. The Midwives Act, 1902; Midwives (Scotland) Act, 1915.
5. Leap and Hunter, *Midwife's Tale*.
6. *Nursing Notes* (January 1928) cited in Leap and Hunter, *Midwife's Tale*, p. 9.
7. Leap and Hunter, *Midwife's Tale*.
8. A. Oakley, *The Captured Womb* (Oxford: Basil Blackwell, 1984).
9. R. Campbell and A. Macfarlane (1994) *Where to Be Born? The Debate and the Evidence*, 2nd edition (Oxford: National Perinatal Epidemiology Unit, 1994).
10. Oakley, *Captured Womb*.
11. Leap and Hunter, *Midwife's Tale*, p. 140.
12. J. Towler and J. Bramall, *Midwives in History and Society* (London: Croom Helm, 1986).
13. J.C. Campbell, *Midwives and Midwifery: Carnegie United Kingdom Trust, Report of the Physical Welfare of Mothers and Children*, vol. 2 (Liverpool: C. Tinling and Co., 1917).
14. A.S. Williams, *Women and Childbirth in the Twentieth Century* (Stroud: Sutton Publishing Ltd, 1997).
15. Leap and Hunter, *Midwife's Tale*.
16. J. Kent, *Social Perspectives on Pregnancy and Childbirth for Midwives, Nurses and the Caring Professions* (Buckingham: Open University Press, 2000).
17. Towler and Bramall, *Midwives*, p. 205.

18. Leap and Hunter, *Midwife's Tale*.
19. Campbell, *Midwives*.
20. Campbell and Macfarlane, *Where to Be Born?*
21. Campbell and Macfarlane, *Where to Be Born?*
22. British Medical Association, 'The BMA and Maternity Services', *British Medical Journal*, 1 (1936) 656.
23. J.C. Campbell, *Reports on Public Health and Medical Subjects: No. 21: The Training of Midwives* (London: HMSO, 1923).
24. Williams, *Women*.
25. Towler and Bramall, *Midwives*.
26. Leap and Hunter, *Midwife's Tale*, p. 55.
27. Towler and Bramall, *Midwives*, p. 226.
28. Leap and Hunter, *Midwife's Tale*, p. 55.
29. Towler and Bramall, *Midwives*.
30. Williams, *Women*.
31. Towler and Bramall, *Midwives*.
32. Leap and Hunter, *Midwife's Tale*.
33. Leap and Hunter, *Midwife's Tale*.
34. Campbell and Macfarlane, *Where to Be Born?* p. 45.
35. Towler and Bramall, *Midwives*, p. 232.
36. Ministry of Health, *The Midwives Salaries Committee*, Rushcliffe Report (London: HMSO, 1943).
37. R. Dingwall, A.M. Rafferty and C. Webster, *An Introduction to the Social History of Nursing* (London: Routledge, 1988) p. 168.
38. Campbell and Macfarlane, *Where to Be Born?*
39. Royal College of Obstetricians and Gynaecologists, *Report on a National Maternity Service* (London: RCOG, 1944).
40. Royal College of Obstetricians and Gynaecologists, *Report on the Obstetric Service under the NHS* (London: RCOG, 1954).
41. L. Durward and R. Evans, 'Pressure Groups and Maternity Care', in J. Garcia, R. Kilpatrick and M. Richards (eds), *The Politics of Maternity Care: Services for Childbearing Women in Twentieth-Century Britain* (Oxford: Oxford University Press, 1990) pp. 256–73.
42. A. Symonds and S.C. Hunt, *The Midwife and Society* (Basingstoke: Macmillan Press, 1996) p. 92.
43. M. Tew, *Safer Childbirth? A Critical History of Maternity Care* (London: Chapman and Hall, 1990).
44. Symonds and Hunt, *Midwife*.
45. J. Sandall, 'Continuity of Midwifery Care in England: A New Professional Project?' *Gender, Work and Organisation*, 3:4 (1990) 215–26.
46. Dingwall, Rafferty and Webster, *Introduction*.
47. Leap and Hunter, *Midwife's Tale*, p. 59.
48. Towler and Bramall, *Midwives*; Tew, *Safer Childbirth?*
49. Campbell and Macfarlane, *Where to Be Born?*; Tew, *Safer Childbirth?*

50. J. Kitzinger, 'Strategies of the Early Childbirth Movement: A Case Study of the National Childbirth Trust', in J. Garcia, R. Kilpatrick and M. Richards (eds), *The Politics of Maternity Care: Services for Childbearing Women in Twentieth-Century Britain* (Oxford: Oxford University Press, 1990) pp. 92–115.

51. *Report of the Committee of Enquiry into the Cost of the National Health Service*, Chairman Lord Guillebaud (London: HMSO, 1956) p. 212.

52. Ministry of Health, *Report of the Maternity Services Committee*, Chairman: Lord Cranbrook (London: HMSO, 1959).

53. Towler and Bramall, *Midwives*.

54. National Birthday Trust Fund, 'Evidence to Maternity Services Committee'. Wellcome Library [WL], SA/NBT/U.11/11: Box 209, 1956.

55. S. Snow and E. Jones, 'Immigration and the NHS: Putting History to the Forefront', *History and Policy*, http://www.historyandpolicy.org/papers/policy-paper-118.html#S6, accessed 5 May 2011.

56. Snow and Jones, 'Immigration'.

57. Royal College of Midwives, 'The Midwife in the Maternity Services', Memorandum to Cranbrook Committee. WL, SA/NBT/U.11/11: Box 209. 1955, p. 3.

58. Royal College of Midwives, *Midwife*, p. 2.

59. Royal College of Midwives, *Midwife*, p. 3.

60. Ministry of Health, *Report of the Maternity Services Committee* cited in Tew, *Safer Childbirth?* p. 154.

61. J.F. Walker, 'Midwife or Obstetric Nurse? Some Perceptions of Midwives and Obstetricians of the Role of the Midwife', *Journal of Advanced Nursing*, 1 (1976) 129–38.

62. Tew, *Safer Childbirth?* p. 154.

63. Campbell and Macfarlane, *Where to Be Born?*

64. Sandall, 'Continuity'.

65. Oakley, *Captured Womb*.

66. Walker, 'Midwife'.

67. Towler and Bramall, *Midwives*, p. 253.

68. Tew, *Safer Childbirth?* p. 67.

69. R.E. Davis-Floyd and C.F. Sargent, *Childbirth and Authoritative Knowledge: Cross-Cultural Perspectives* (Berkeley, California: University of California Press, 1997).

70. Standing Maternity and Midwifery Advisory Committee, *Domiciliary Midwifery and Maternity Bed Needs*, Chairman: J. Peel (London: HMSO, 1970) p. 60.

71. G.W. Lewis and P. McCaffery, 'Sociological Factors Affecting the Medicalization of Midwifery', in E. Van Teijlingen, G. Lowis, P. McCaffery and M. Porter (eds), *Midwifery and the Medicalization of Childbirth: Comparative Perspectives* (New York: Nova Science Publishers, 2000) pp. 5–41.

72. Percival, 'Management', p. 204.
73. M. Kirkham, 'Labouring in the Dark: Limitations on the Giving of Information to Enable Patients to Orientate Themselves to the Likely Events and Timescale of Labour', in J. Wilson-Barnett (ed.), *Nursing Research: Ten Studies in Patient Care* (Chichester: Wiley, 1983) pp. 81–99.
74. Sandall, 'Continuity'.
75. Dingwall, Rafferty and Webster, *Introduction*, p. 171.
76. K. O'Driscoll, D. Meagher and P. Boylan, *Active Management of Labour* (London: Mosby, 1993).
77. Davis-Floyd and Sargent, *Childbirth*.
78. R.G. DeVries, 'A Cross-National View of the Status of Midwives', in E. Riska and K. Wegar (eds), *Gender, Work and Medicine: Women and the Medical Division of Labour* (London: Sage, 1993) pp. 131–46.
79. Towler and Bramall, *Midwives*, p. 271.
80. D. Haire, *The Cultural Warping of Childbirth* (Wisconsin, USA: International Childbirth Education Association, 1972); M. Odent, *Entering the World. The De-Medicalisation of Childbirth* (London: Marion Boyars, 1984).
81. S. Kitzinger (ed.), *Episiotomy: Physical and Emotional Aspects* (London: National Childbirth Trust, 1981).
82. S. Kitzinger, *The Midwife Challenge* (London: Pandora, 1988) p. 18.
83. R. Weitz, 'English Midwives and the Association of Radical Midwives', *Women and Health*, 12:1 (1987) 79–89.
84. Weitz, 'English Midwives'.
85. Association of Radical Midwives, *The Role of the Midwife*, Conference Report of the Association of Radical Midwives, First Annual Conference on the Role of the Midwife, June 1981, Sheffield (London: ARM, 1981).
86. Weitz, 'English Midwives'.
87. Weitz, 'English Midwives', p. 88.
88. Association of Radical Midwives, *The Vision: Proposals for the Future of the Maternity Services* (Ormskirk: ARM, 1986).
89. United Kingdom Central Council for Nursing, Midwifery and Health Visiting, *Project 2000: A New Preparation for Practice* (London: UKCC, 1986).
90. Kent, *Social Perspectives*.
91. M. Cronk, 'Midwifery: A Practitioner's View from within the National Health Services', *Midwife, Health Visitor and Community Nurse*, 26:3 (1990) 58–63.
92. Association of Radical Midwives, *Vision*.
93. Department of Health, *Working for Patients: Education and Training*, Working Paper 10 (London: HMSO, 1989).
94. House of Commons Select Committee, *Second Report: Maternity Services* (London: HMSO, 1992).

95. Department of Health (1993) *Changing Childbirth: Part 1: Report of the Expert Maternity Group* (London: HMSO, 1993) p. 8.
96. Welsh Health Planning Forum, *Protocol for Investment in Health Gain, Maternal and Early Child Health* (Cardiff: Welsh Office NHS Directorate, 1991).
97. Tew, *Safer Childbirth?*
98. I. Chalmers, M. Enkin and M.J.N.C. Keirse, *Effective Care in Pregnancy and Childbirth* (Oxford: Oxford University Press, 1989).
99. M. Porter, 'Changing Childbirth? The British Midwife's Role in Research and Innovation', in Van Teijlingen, Lowis, McCaffery and Porter (eds), *Midwifery*, pp. 183–93.
100. J. Sandall, 'Choice, Continuity and Control: Changing Midwifery, towards a Sociological Perspective', *Midwifery*, 11 (1995) 201–9.
101. Department of Health, *Changing Childbirth*, p. 16.
102. L. Long, 'Changing Childbirth: Views and Comment. Implications for Clinical Midwives at Grass Roots Level', *British Journal of Midwifery*, 1:5 (1993) 231; L. Page, 'Changing Childbirth', *Modern Midwife* (November/December 1993) 28–9.
103. J. Schott, 'Changing Childbirth: Views and Comment. Changing Ourselves', *British Journal of Midwifery*, 1:5 (1999) 230; R. Clarke, 'Normal Services Will Be Resumed?' *Modern Midwife* (December 1994) 36–7.
104. Department of Health, *Maternity Matters: Choice, Access and Continuity of Care in a Safe Service* (London: DoH, 2007).
105. Williams, *Women*.
106. Kent, *Social Perspectives*.
107. C. Rees, 'A Retrospective: Jennifer Sleep's Classic Research Study on the Use of Episiotomy in Labour', *MIDIRS Midwifery Digest*, 17:3 (2007) 319–22.

PART III

COMPARING NURSING AND MIDWIFERY

The final part of the book consists of three chapters which compare nursing and midwifery, taking account of the influence of social, political and cultural contexts.

In Chapter 8: *International Comparisons: The Nursing–Midwifery Interface*, Winifred Connerton and Patricia D'Antonio provide an international comparison by considering the respective – and very different – histories of nursing and midwifery in three well-resourced countries: Australia, the United States and Canada. The authors analyse how the practice of nursing and midwifery, and the boundary between the two professions, has been historically shaped by the influence of the United Kingdom and the United States. Connerton and D'Antonio focus on how the professionalizing project of nurses in all three countries has affected the work of midwives, observing that, in the countries they discuss, the rise in the status of professional nursing has been directly linked to the decreased status of midwifery practice.

In Chapter 9: *Nursing and Midwifery: An Uneasy Alliance or Natural Bedfellows?*, Billie Hunter and Anne Borsay continue the exploration of the interface between nursing and midwifery, throwing light on the interprofessional tensions and 'tribalism' which are often described. Focusing on UK health care, the authors provide a comparative analysis of nursing and midwifery history, exploring the ways in which the two professions can be considered similar or divergent, and examining the conflicts and allegiances which have emerged and continue to exist. They draw attention to the complexity of the relationship and the key themes which need considering in order for it to be better understood: occupational autonomy, specificity of role, professional boundaries, relationships with medical practitioners and professionalization strategies.

In the final chapter: *Epilogue: Contemporary Challenges,* Jane Sandall and Anne Marie Rafferty bring the discussion up to the present day by considering what the 'lessons of history' offer contemporary nurses and midwives as they encounter the challenges of the twenty-first century. Arguing from their perspective as sociologists of health care, they propose that there are a number of enduring themes in the histories of nursing and midwifery, so that there is more in common with past challenges than any radical divergence. By investigating the histories of the respective professions, new insights into current problems can be gained.

8

International Comparisons: The Nursing–Midwifery Interface

Winifred Connerton and Patricia D'Antonio

The world of nursing and midwifery has been historically shaped by two global (and sometimes competing) spheres of influence: that of the United Kingdom and that of the United States. The United Kingdom and some of its colonies developed a model that included nursing and midwifery as parallel professions. Midwifery had long been an acceptable and respected form of post-registration practice for nursing, with that role existing easily alongside nursing roles such as district nursing and health visiting. Simultaneously, the United Kingdom had a long tradition of direct-entry midwifery. Both nurse trained and direct-entry midwives were registered by the same regulatory body, were governed by the same rules and standards and could belong to the same professional organization, the Royal College of Midwives (RCM). They worked together throughout the twentieth century, to establish a strong political base that they successfully used to set educational standards and to protect the independence of their practice.

In contrast, in the United States, as in some of the British colonies such as Australia and Canada, direct-entry midwives had no such organizations and the twentieth-century legitimation of their practice took much longer to establish. Relationships with nurse-midwives were more tentative. Indeed, many nurses in the United States and its colonies and protectorates supported the medical professionalization

177

of obstetrics, concentrating instead on developing post-graduate public health nurses who would work for health and welfare programmes related to the care of mothers and children. Nurses in these roles initially joined medical colleagues in pushing for the elimination of midwifery – a form of practice which, unlike that in the United Kingdom, was associated primarily with poor, immigrant and African-American women. Yet, whatever the educational and professional background of these midwives and nurse-midwives, they all shared a commonality of practice: the private and intimate care that existed at the birthing woman's bedside. As such, personal preferences, local norms, historical traditions and deeply held beliefs also shaped practices.

This chapter looks specifically at the history of nurse–midwifery interface, paying particular attention to the effects on the work of midwives as nursing engaged in its own professionalizing project. It considers midwifery practices as situated at the intersection of the global and the local; and midwives themselves as part of an international movement to increase standardization, training and practices that best served unique communities of women with their own culture and systems of authority. We begin when traditional practices of midwifery in the form of 'granny midwives' and handywomen had begun to give way to those which required certain forms of credentials. Historically, many different kinds of women and men with many different backgrounds and different learning experiences have laid claim to the practice of midwifery. To add clarity to the process of naming each kind of practice, we have adopted the definitions that follow. We consider a lay midwife as one who practised without formal training, usually within her own community. These midwives were also known as granny midwives, handywomen and traditional birth attendants. Qualifications for lay midwifery included being a woman and, often, having borne children of one's own. Generally these midwives operated within a community network based on location, ethnicity, religion and class. Although known to their own communities, there was little to no formal recognition of their practice, and no certification or licensure system available for them. We define trained midwives as those women who had received formal training for the care and delivery of pregnant women. Very early in this period, training would have been by apprenticeship; by the mid to late nineteenth century, formal training programmes, often associated with hospitals, were being established specifically for training midwives. In the United States and the United Kingdom, these midwives became known as direct-entry midwives. Nurse-midwives, by contrast, had first trained as general nurses and then received midwifery training as part of a post-graduate programme in nursing. These midwives attended training programmes that considered midwifery as a branch of nursing rather than as an independent profession; and received formal certification to practice.

The history of twentieth-century British nursing and midwifery, discussed in detail in Chapters 4 and 7, has been highly influential in what we now consider to be modern nursing and midwifery practice. We will examine how the British sphere of influence affected the development of these professions in Australia and consider the adaptability of the British model to different social, political and professional contexts. We then contrast this with an exploration of the interface between nursing and midwifery in the United States before considering the development of midwifery in Canada, a country which looked to traditions from both the United Kingdom and the United States. All three countries are well resourced and well researched. The chapter adopts a comparative approach. While local particularities and individual agency may be lost, looking beyond traditional nation-state boundaries helps us to locate and understand cross-cutting influences. As Stephan Berger has argued, 'No other historical method is so adept at testing, modifying and falsifying historical explanation as comparison.'[1]

Australia

The evolution of trained nursing and midwifery in Australia is a story of overlapping professions, neither one entirely separate from the other, and yet neither lying comfortably together. Australia was first settled by the British in 1788. Australia's white settlers were varied in their reasons for emigration and in their backgrounds. For example, the territories of Eastern Australia were established in part as convict settlements, while Southern Australia was founded with the intention of long-term settlement and colonial expansion.[2] These settlements developed into individual states with their own systems for the regulation of nursing and midwifery care and education. Across Australia professional midwifery, nursing and medicine developed together, with nursing aligning with medicine to achieve professional status and, until very recently, midwifery achieving a symbiotic relationship with nursing rather than professional independence.

The first nurses and midwives in Australia came on the ships bringing convicts to the settlements – they were simply other convicts or servants with an inclination or assignment to care for their fellow travellers.[3] Lesley Barclay has termed the initial midwifery services available in the convict colonies as 'accidental midwifery', when assistance in childbirth came from whoever may have been available, followed by the 'Aunt Rubina period' when older, married female relations or neighbours came to help younger women in childbirth.[4] The midwifery care in these periods involved untrained midwives; it was not until 1824 that trained midwifery came to Tasmania along with waves of colonists.[5] Trained nursing also came from abroad with the arrival of Nightingale nurses from London at the Sydney Infirmary in 1868.[6] Previously, hospitals existed as charitable institutions for the destitute, and as part of the administration of the penal colony, and nursing care was rendered by untrained practitioners who were usually men or catholic nursing sisters.[7] Trained midwives and nurses changed the health-care landscape. Neighbour midwives and untrained male nurses were eventually replaced by their trained competitors. Though untrained midwifery persisted for longer than untrained nursing, it was eventually subsumed into a division of nursing practice.

The regional differences in midwifery care throughout Australia were the result of the variety of settlement populations in the colony.[8] Annette Summers has noted that once colonization with the intent of permanent settlement began in Australia, the need for competent care in childbirth was essential to expanding the white-settler population.[9] While the local network of lay midwives flourished, trained midwives were also arriving from Britain and establishing practices in the new colony.[10] The first Australian midwifery training programme was at the Melbourne Lying-In Hospital in 1862, and others developed as the population grew with the first programme in South Australia beginning in 1902 at the Queen's Home.[11] These training programmes never graduated enough trained midwives to meet the needs of childbearing women, however, and lay midwifery continued without any restriction until the beginning of the twentieth century when the state of Tasmania instituted Australia's first regulation of midwives with the 1901 Midwifery Act.[12]

Midwives still had active state support in rural regions where few health-care providers existed, but the decline of midwifery as an independent profession in urban locales began in the early twentieth century as nursing and medicine began to encroach on traditional midwifery practice.[13] State interest in childbearing intersected with midwifery regulation in Victoria, where the government instituted a 'baby bonus' programme to boost the white population in 1912.

Initially midwife-attended births were included in the programme, but by 1922 it was only medically attended births that qualified for the bonus.[14] A Midwife Registration Bill establishing a Midwife Board to oversee trained midwifery passed through Parliament in 1915, but in 1928 the Board was eliminated and midwives were brought into the sphere of nursing.[15] Summers notes that the extent of lay midwives practising throughout the colonies was evidenced when the Nurses' Act was passed and those midwives began writing to the Board seeking to comply with registration requirements.[16] The development of trained nursing education and registration meant the beginning of the end for lay midwives, and a shift away from independence for trained midwives.

The nursing training also shifted the understanding of what it meant to nurse the sick. Prior to the Nightingale nurses, nursing in hospitals was done by men. These men did not receive any special training, and in fact, with the advent of trained nursing, men were pushed out of the field in favour of the 'ladies' that conformed to the Nightingale model of a nursing caregiver. Judith Godden has written extensively on Lucy Osburn, the British nurse who brought Nightingale nursing to Australia.[17] The Sydney Infirmary and Dispensary (later the Sydney Hospital) was run by the New South Wales government for impoverished free citizens. As Godden recounts, the physicians of the hospital and its Board of Directors had long advocated for improved nursing care at the hospital, but it was not until a well-publicized death of a paying patient that the government was forced to approve the expense of employing trained nurses.[18] Lucy Osburn's legacy is the introduction of trained nursing to Australia as many nurses from her training programme went on to found other hospitals' training schools.[19] Even more, though, the legacy of trained nursing in Australia was the change from untrained work done by convicts, servants and uneducated people to a profession of 'ladies' that required education.[20]

Lavinia Dock, American nursing leader and editor of the *American Journal of Nursing's* 'Foreign Department' trumpeted the 1899 formation of the Australasian Trained Nurses' Association (ATNA), and quoted Miss S.B. McGahey's explanation of what the association would do for Australian nurses:

> The Australasian Trained Nurses' Association is daily becoming better known, and it is hoped before many years have elapsed that the medical profession and the public who employ nurses will have only

those who are properly trained, and thereby stamp out the untrained women who style themselves nurses and flourish in the Australasian colonies.[21]

Though the founding of the ATNA was first a meeting of like-minded professional nurses and physicians, the Association rapidly began working for legislation and regulation of the profession. In 1906 they held their first examination for (voluntary) national registration, and by 1927 each of the states had nursing boards and requirements of registration for practice.[22] Nursing education remained in hospitals until the 1970s when the first university programmes opened.[23] The association of nursing with formal education helped change the understanding of what made a qualified health practitioner. No longer was it acceptable to have the servant or neighbour offer nursing services in the home or hospital.

This same culture shift affected midwifery as well. Historians of midwifery have argued that Australian midwifery never developed as a fully independent profession for multiple reasons, including active suppression by the medical community and nursing's collusion with medicine against midwifery to gain more professional power. Lesley Barclay has noted that midwives did not have any professional organization to defend attacks on their profession from the medical community. She writes 'midwives were neither powerful nor organized as a group to resist. Married women, constrained by the demands of their own families, lack of funds and education, did not really constitute any opposition to medicine's take over.'[24] Summers has suggested that medicine is to blame for the midwives' incorporation into nursing because 'The only way that medicine could have any control over midwifery was through nursing.'[25] Fiona Bogossian notes that the lack of strong midwifery advocates made midwifery's subordination to nursing a 'foregone conclusion'.[26] She goes on to argue that across Australia each of the states situated midwifery under the umbrella of nursing from the beginning of training and registration. Some regions did allow for the registration of midwives who were not nurses, though this was irregular and infrequent. Although there was nominal midwifery presence within registration legislation and administration, Bogossian notes that there was no place set aside for midwives on the regulatory boards and, consequently, no one defending midwifery's individual interests.[27] For midwifery in the early twentieth century, the advent of trained nursing, increasing power of physicians and hospital directors, and women's changing expectations of being attended by a trained provider created the perfect storm for the submersion of midwifery into nursing.

This confluence of trained nursing and midwifery came about, in part, because of the training and regulatory process. For example, in Melbourne there was an existing midwifery training programme at the Women's Hospital. Trained nurses came to Melbourne in 1871, a city that wanted to improve its care along the lines of the Sydney Infirmary by introducing trained nurses in the Nightingale mould.[28] By 1893 the programme was restricted to graduate nurses, with midwifery now limited to training as a midwifery nurse, one who worked under a physician's supervision.[29] The ATNA also helped combine nursing and midwifery. ATNA was founded in 1899 and trained midwives who were also nurses were granted membership in the nursing Register. Trained midwives who were not nurses, however, were granted ATNA membership, but with special restrictions. For example, it was only the nurse-midwives among the ATNA who could vote within the organization, and the general council, the central organizing committee within ATNA, had no midwifery representation at all.[30] The Nurses Registration Act of South Australia in 1920 was the first legislation which explicitly linked midwifery to nursing registration. This Act, which created the licensure of nurses in the state, also made care by unregistered midwives illegal, and eventually under this legislation midwifery in Australia became obstetric nursing rather than an independent profession.[31]

Midwifery did not completely disappear, but until recently the only route to trained midwifery practice in Australia was through nursing as a post-graduate specialization.[32] Today trained midwifery in Australia is regulated under each state's nursing registration board and the Australian College of Midwives is the umbrella professional organization. After almost a century of training in nursing schools, the option of direct-entry education for midwifery was re-instated in 1999 in the form of a three-year Bachelor's degree of midwifery without a previous nursing degree.[33] The re-emergence of direct-entry trained midwifery was due to a combination of frustration by trained midwives with their limited scope of practice, and community-led advocacy for different birthing options for pregnant women.[34] The numbers of direct-entry trained midwives in Australia are still small, and there is some evidence that graduates find their advancement limited by lack of a nursing degree necessary for further academic study.[35] Trained midwifery in Australia reflected the colonial and national interest in safe childbearing. By providing safe obstetric care in remote areas, and later by participating in the baby bonus programmes, mid-wives were seen by the government as a useful access point into families' lives until more centralized care services were established. This was true in the United States as well.

United States

In the United States, formally trained nurses saw the opening decades of the twentieth century as a critical time that held significant possibilities as well as long simmering problems. In 1890, there were still fewer than 500 trained nurses across the country, but the numbers of trained nurses grew rapidly to 3,500 in 1900 and over 8,000 in 1910.[36] Significant issues had emerged. There was wide variation in training experiences. Hospitals controlled the training schools, and the curricular content and experiences varied widely. Some graduates of the larger, more prosperous, urban hospital-based training schools received excellent training, particularly in the five areas of practice which leading nursing educationalists believed to be critical: medical, surgical, obstetrics, paediatrics and dietetics. However, others who trained in smaller, specialized or rural units which were some-times resource-starved had a more limited experience. Nonetheless, after training, they were held in high esteem and became among the more educated and respected members of either the urban or rural communities from which they came.[37]

All these nurses shared a strong nursing identity and commitment to practice. They also shared an abiding faith in the promise offered by the newly emerging scientific medicine and a strong belief in the value of its particular practices. As Patricia D'Antonio has argued, early twentieth-century medical knowledge had yet to produce the thrilling achievements that would mirror that seen in surgical and public health practices. But its foundations were in science and its learning was in a hospital. In these new public spaces, nurses, predominantly female, drew on this new scientific knowledge to enhance their authority and standing. This was particularly important when challenged by families who claimed personalized and subjective knowledge. Most of these challenges came after graduation when the vast majority of trained nurses took positions as private duty nurses. These nurses left the hospital environment to work in the private homes of families who employed them, as homes were still the preferred site for the treatment of illnesses and caring for sick individuals. Some eventually returned to hospitals, becoming operating room nurses as surgery in hospitals became more prominent, or head nurses, supervisors or directors of training schools teaching the next generation of nurses. And an even smaller number entered the field of public health nursing – one of the most prestigious and independent fields of nursing practice.[38]

Public health nursing was born in the late nineteenth-century movement to provide care to the sick poor in their own homes. In larger and more urban areas across the United States, wealthy philanthropists provided the monies to send a private duty nurse, soon called a visiting nurse, into the homes of those who could not afford one. As Karen Buhler-Wilkerson has argued, this generosity arose from multiple and complicated motives.[39] Some of those in need of care were native born, but many were newly arrived immigrants (on the east coast: western and southern Europe; on the west coast: China and Japan) who needed both care and a gentle introduction to the norms of American society as well as its health and healing practices. They needed, in Buhler-Wilkerson's words, both 'medicine and a message'.[40] But even as these philanthropists and nurses sought to help others, they also felt they needed to protect themselves. New knowledge about what was known as the 'germ theory' had slipped from the laboratory into the public discourse. Some of the implications seemed frightening: it was no longer enough to control one's own health habits and practices, one also had to control those of others lest their germs travel and infect innocent bystanders. Others seemed exhilarating: knowledge about germ transmission was growing day-by-day and the emerging science of public health promised effective practices that would halt germ transmission and promote healthy lifestyles.[41]

In the opening decades of the twentieth century, public health nursing practices stood at the centre of these complicated and sometimes conflicting motives. Unlike visiting nurses who cared for the sick at home, public health nurses joined campaigns to tackle the most vexing issues affecting the health of individuals and communities. They were on the front line of efforts to prevent the transmission of tuberculosis, one of the leading causes of death during this period, and to identify and send into treatment those with active infections. They were very active in work to reduce maternal and infant mortality by promoting prenatal care, breastfeeding, good nutrition and clean (non-infected with bovine tuberculosis) milk. And they joined with physicians to tackle the issue that was then widely known as the 'midwife problem'.[42]

Lay midwifery, in the United States and across the globe, had its roots in practices of experienced women helping other women in childbirth and the post-partum period. Laurel Thatcher Ulrich paints a rich portrait of the life of one such early midwife, Martha Ballard, drawing on the diaries she kept between 1785 and 1812 to show how a life as a midwife was intricately connected to a simultaneous life as a wife, mother, nurse and respected community member. For example, on 18th November 1793 after attending her 48th birth that year, Martha Ballard records:

> At Capt Melloys. His lady in Labour. Her women Calld (it was a sever storm of rain Cleard of with snow). My patient deliverd at 8 hour 5 minute Evening of a fine daughter. Her attendants wrre Mrss Cleark, Duttun, Sewall, & myself. We had an Elligant supper and I tarried all night.[43]

Ballard, like other midwives throughout the country, concentrated her practice within her immediate, albeit large, geographic area and, when necessary, consulted with a neighbouring physician. But Ballard, again like other midwives throughout the country, had more experience than that physician in delivering infants.

Through much of the nineteenth century, midwives like Ballard delivered most infants in the United States. The only exception was the socially prominent, native born, white urban women who often chose a physician as their birth attendant. But, in similar ways, the choice of a particular midwife birth attendant reflected the same issues of class, geography, ethnicity and race among different groups of women. African-American and Native American women turned to their own lay midwives in childbirth, and communities of immigrants to the United States always included among their numbers their own midwives. Some, like the mid-nineteenth century Irish immigrants, included lay midwives who had learned their practices through experience. Others, such as later immigrants from central Europe and Japan, had already trained in formal, state-regulated midwifery programmes.[44] They often acted as, in Susan Smith's words, 'culture brokers', helping other women in their communities integrate norms of their home countries with those of their new one and holding the respect of their own particular communities.[45] Irrespective of backgrounds, though, those with some formal training achieved birth outcomes as good as if not better than physicians.[46]

Yet despite their achievements and status within the community, by the turn of the twentieth century these African-American and immigrant midwives also experienced the suspicions and sometimes the scorn of more affluent white physicians, nurses and public health officials.[47] This attitude was underpinned by a new 'scientific' approach to childbirth. The ascendency of scientific medicine and nursing, with its new understanding of the implications of laboratory science and disease transmission, brought with it a standardization of educational training and credentialing. It also brought with it a profound optimism that problematic issues of health and illness could be solved. One of the more pressing problems was that of unacceptably high maternal and infant mortality rates. From this perspective, midwifery, with its complicated matrix of race, class and gender, appeared to lack standardization and a scientific knowledge base. At best, it was considered ill-informed, and, at worst, dangerous and shrouded in superstition.[48] As a result, physician-led births became the ideal. Local departments of public health undertook an ambitious goal to have every birth experience of American mothers attended by a physician. This was later supported by the United States Government's 1921 Sheppard-Towner Act (which provided federal support for female physicians and public health nurses to care for women and infants), and the federal Children's Bureau (which provided education to mothers about the best ways to care for their infants and families). In areas such as the rural South where the shortage of physicians remained problematic the goal would be to temporarily use public health nurses to systematically train midwives in new techniques of infection control and then to carefully supervise them to ensure they incorporated such techniques into their practices.

Not surprisingly, the numbers of midwife-attended births dropped dramatically throughout the early decades of the twentieth century as women turned to physician-attended and later hospital-based births. But, as Judith Leavitt points out, it was not a simple process of professional control and dominance.[49] Birthing women themselves were the most active agents of change. Native-born white women were the ones seeking the perceived safety, pain control and protection that a more scientific approach to childbirth promised. And they were swiftly followed by daughters of immigrants and those African-American families able to access medical resources, who turned away from traditional midwife-attended births in their quest to access the same services available to white middle-class women. The numbers of midwife-attended births continued to plummet in the United States – until by the mid-1950s most births were attended by doctors, with labour and delivery nurses in a supporting role.

Yet, the issue of high maternal and infant mortality rates remained stubbornly high. Clearly, physician-led birth was not the answer. In response, some public health nurses turned to the British model of midwifery training, certification and supervision created by the Midwives' Act of 1902. With the support of prominent American foundations, such as the Rockefeller and the Kellogg Foundations, they tentatively experimented with the idea of training nurses as midwives. In New York City, home to some of the most progressive public health nursing initiatives, an initiative was set in motion by the Maternity Care Association, one of the leading (and successful) private organizations dedicated to using public health nurses to reduce the high maternal and infant mortality rates. The Association attempted to build links to leading hospital nurse training schools, with the ultimate aim of establishing a school for nurse-midwives. It struggled for decades, trying to convince physicians that nurse-midwives would not compete with them for patients and trying to convince nurses that practicing as nurse-midwives would not conflate their work with that of the widely disparaged lay midwives.[50] It finally succeeded with the establishment of the privately funded Lobenstine Midwifery Clinic in 1931 and the Lobenstine Midwifery School in 1932. The Clinic and School's scope was limited and the number of graduates who ultimately practiced as nurse-midwives was very small. The only opportunities to practice were on medical religious missions. Most graduates returned to public health or hospital practices where they supervised nurses in pre- and post-natal care.[51]

Mary Breckinridge had more success with her Frontier Nursing Service (FNS), which used nurse-midwives to serve the women in Kentucky's rural mountains. Breckinridge, a member of a socially and politically prominent American family, found her way first to nursing and then to midwifery through a series of devastating personal losses (including the deaths of her two children) and experiences as a relief worker in France after the First World War. As recounted in *Wide Neighborhoods,* her autobiography and fund-raising tool, there she witnessed the success of and respect for British nurse-midwives.[52] As there was no nurse-midwife training available in the United States, Breckinridge travelled to London in 1923 to study at the British Hospital for Mothers and Babies. She subsequently established the FNS in 1925, staffed by American nurse-midwives who she had sent to the United Kingdom for training and British nurse-midwives she successfully recruited to Kentucky.

The FNS soon proved successful – at both meeting the birthing and health needs of Kentucky's women and being financially viable. The money needed for its operations was raised from donors across the United States who were fascinated by pictures of nurse-midwives on horseback as they found their way to remote mountain cabins to deliver babies. But the outbreak of the Second World War threatened the FNS's services. British nurse-midwives returned home to work in their own country and it became difficult, if not impossible, to send American nurses abroad to train. In response, the FNS began its own school for nurse-midwives in 1939, a school that still trains nurse-midwives today.[53]

The Second World War also affected the work of the Medical Mission Sisters, a Catholic nursing order that had focused its work abroad. Finding themselves restricted to the United States, the order accepted an invitation to battle the extremely high rates of infant mortality in Santa Fe, New Mexico. Two of its members were sent to first train as nurse-midwives at the Lobenstine Midwifery School in New York City, and then, in 1944, to open the Catholic Maternity Institute (CMI) to both serve birthing women and continue to train other sister nurses as nurse-midwives. The CMI had a different history than the FNS. The nurse-midwives had opened *La Casita,* a free-standing building where mothers who lived at a considerable distance could come to give birth. Over time, mothers preferred the more expensive option of *La Casita* births to home births, and, as expenses mounted, the Medical Mission Sisters decided its slim economic resources would be best used by returning to their pre-Second World War commitment to work abroad. The CMI closed in 1969.[54]

The practice of nurse-midwifery grew slowly in the United States. But in the second half of the century an increasing birthrate, a shortage of obstetricians and an increasing wish by middle-class American mothers to have more control over their birthing experience drew more and more nurses into midwifery training. By 1954, the numbers of nurses identifying as nurse-midwives were sufficient enough to form the new American College of Nurse-Midwives (ACNM). But self-identifying and practicing were two quite separate matters. Only 11 of the approximately 400 nurse-midwives actually practiced clinical midwifery.[55] Most of the early members of the ACNM actually practiced as nursing educators, administrators or consultants to maternal and child health programmes rather than as 'hands-on' nurse-midwives.[56]

Concomitantly, white middle-class mothers who wanted an alternative birth experience began turning away from nurse-midwives, whom they believed were complicit with the medical model of childbirth, and towards lay midwives. Although the actual numbers were never very large, the demand for lay midwives was strong enough for the ACNM to begin an accreditation process for schools of midwifery for direct-entry midwives. These graduates would sit an ACNM certification examination, and, on its successful completion, become Certified Midwives (also called direct-entry midwives) with full membership rights to the ACNM.[57]

Numbers of direct-entry midwives remain small and difficult to quantify; and their numbers include those whose formal training ranges from none, to apprenticeships, to formal post-baccalaureate programmes in midwifery. Tensions remain between the ACNM, whose membership includes direct-entry midwives from schools it accredits, and a newer organization, the Midwives Alliance of North America (MANA), created in 1982 as an umbrella group of all midwives, including direct-entry midwives from formal training programmes not accredited by the ACNM. Regulatory oversight varies from place to place: in some states midwifery falls under the jurisdiction of state Boards of Medicine; in others under state Boards of Nursing. And the relationship between nursing and midwifery still remains a work-in-progress: are nurse-midwives nurses with a specialty practice; or is midwifery a practice independent of nursing?

The effects are still experienced today. Numbers of direct-entry midwives remain small. Whereas nurse-midwives and midwives deliver 80 per cent of infants world-wide, they deliver less that 11 per cent in the United States. As Katy Dawley has wryly noted, the early twentieth-century attack on the 'midwife problem' worked all too well.[58]

Canada

Nursing and midwifery in Canada carry the legacy of Canada's unique colonial origins. France, as the first colonial presence, was responsible for the earliest nursing and midwifery services for colonial populations, with Catholic nursing sisters offering care in the Quebec *Hotel Dieu* as well as community-based midwife services furnished by local governments.[59] The later integration of the French system with the developing British model in the other colonies resulted in the promotion of public health nursing over midwifery. However, midwifery in

Canada was never fully outlawed, rather it suffered from government's benign neglect and, in some cases, its tacit approval.

The first permanent French settlement in North America was at Port Royal in 1605 as part of the fur trade. Veronica Strong-Boag has chronicled the evolution of nursing in Canada from its earliest days in Roman Catholic hospitals and missions. In New France colonists enjoyed health care similar to that in France itself. The first hospitals were opened in 1639 in the form of Roman Catholic medical missions to the First Nation people in Quebec and Montreal. One of these, the *Hotel Dieu,* also ran a training school for hospital attendants. This was not a formal nursing training programme based on scientific education, but an apprentice model of instruction in care of the sick.[60] Other hospitals soon followed, and what is now Quebec province had public health programmes with visiting health attendants, training programmes in hospitals in the larger cities and midwives to attend births throughout the region.[61] Until formal nursing training was introduced by Nightingale nurses in the 1870s, trained and lay midwives offered maternity care throughout the provinces.

Midwifery services in colonial Canadian communities were made up of a combination of trained and lay midwives and physicians, each with a specific scope of practice. Helene Laforce, historian of midwifery in Quebec, explains that under the French midwives were hired into salaried positions to serve the childbearing needs of the entire community. These trained midwives were recruited directly from France where they received their training at the *Hotel Dieu de Paris.* It was sometimes the childbearing women of a community who voted to chose their midwifery providers, and as Laforce notes, this practice allowed women an important role in their own childbirth care.[62] Once the British took administrative control over the French territories, the British medical establishment encountered a population completely accepting midwifery services together with a long-established pattern of 'foreign' educated midwives serving the local population. The existing French system continued well into the nineteenth century with the cooperation of local physicians. In fact, the medical community was so comfortable with midwifery that it was nearly a century before changing medical practice began to displace midwifery in Francophone Canada.[63]

Wendy Mitchinson, in her history of childbirth in Canada, details the development of midwifery outside of French Canada. Mitchinson notes that white-settler women relied not only on their white-settler neighbours but also on First Nation women and midwives for help in labour. Mitchinson also presents evidence that native birthing practices were adopted by settler populations in Newfoundland communities, where white women began giving birth kneeling on the floor in a birth practice similar to that of the native population.[64] Similarly, Cheryl Warsh has detailed how white settlers on the prairies looked to their neighbours for assistance in labour; neighbours who may not have had any experience with birth beyond their own childbearing, as well as to those with experience as trained nurses or midwives.[65] The Canadian Department of Health, understanding that women were far from health providers, issued a special supplement to their publication for mothers, *Canadian Mother's Book*, that gave explicit information about managing a childbirth – essentially a handbook of midwifery.[66]

First Nation midwives could not prevent the toll that disease and displacement took on their communities during the colonial occupation, and by the mid-nineteenth century their populations were dwindling. Missionaries established clinics in far northern First Nation communities, staffed by non-indigenous nurses and physicians, which pushed native midwives and birth practices to the margins.[67] Health provision continued in this manner with untrained nursing attendants and both trained and untrained midwives, until the late nineteenth century, when trained nursing was introduced in Ontario. Midwifery began to decline in this same period as a result of competition and displacement by public nursing services and by conflict with a more organized medical profession.

Trained nursing in Canada developed at about the same time as nursing in Australia and the United States, and its nursing superintendents and leaders came from outside Canada. The first nurse Canadian training school for nursing was St Catharine's (later called the Mack school) in Ontario, established in 1874. This hospital-based school, like its successors at the Montreal General Hospital (1874) and the Toronto General Hospital (1881), had nursing superintendents trained in Britain in the Nightingale model, or trained in the United States.[68] Women interested in nursing also travelled to the United States for their training, and, as Susan Reverby notes, in Boston training schools at the turn of the twentieth century Canadian nursing students represented the largest minority group because of the scarcity of training schools in Canada itself.[69] Quickly, though, Canada became a source for nursing leaders in the United States. Isabelle Hampton Robb and Adelaide Nutting, for example, were both Canadian-born leaders of US nursing.[70] The close affiliation of US nursing leaders with their Canadian peers led to their joint affiliation in the earliest nursing associations. The Association of Superintendents and the Nurses' Associated Alumnae Association both were joint associations of American and Canadian nurses whose members were among the leaders of the profession in both countries. Trained nursing began as a feature of urban hospitals, but public health nursing in Canada spread to the homesteaders in the sparsely populated prairies through a project of the Council of Women.

Nanci Langford has written about women's experiences of childbirth on the prairies, and described their birth experiences as those that 'captured the essence of all that was bad and good about homestead life'.[71] It was out of concern for the infant and maternal mortality of childbearing women on homesteads that the Council of Women, led by Lady Aberdeen, officially known as Ishbel Maria Hamilton-Gordon, Marchioness of Aberdeen and Temair and wife of Canada's Governor General, initiated the Victorian Order of Nurses for Canada (VON) in 1897. As a public health nursing scheme the nurses were not to practice midwifery, rather they would refer childbearing women to local physicians for their births. This made the project palatable to the local medical community who opposed the introduction of a formal midwifery service that would create competition for obstetric cases. The trained nurses on the prairies, however, were not enough to meet the needs of the settlers, and in 1916 the VON again suggested trained midwives for the region. However, this plan was rejected by physicians and the now-formed Nurses Association of Canada who worked to separate trained nursing from any association with midwifery care.[72] Throughout Canada, trained nursing moved from private duty to hospital-based care with a system of public health services for poor urbanites and people in remote regions.

The Canadian government began offering health-care services to First Nation peoples in the early twentieth century as a precautionary manoeuvre to avoid their spreading disease to white-settler populations.[73] The Department of Indian Affairs' Indian Health Service (IHS) provided travelling physicians and dentists as well as local dispensers and field matrons, but these local personnel were not required to have any health service training. However, this system of medical coverage failed at reducing infant mortality and preventing infectious diseases like tuberculosis, and in 1953 the health services were transferred to the Department of National Health and Welfare (DNHW). The DNHW started a system of hospitals, nursing stations and community health centres, which were very successful. Kathryn

McPherson has detailed the ways that these health services continued a colonial relationship between the government and First Nation communities, even while they also created an effective system of health services. Beginning with field matrons teaching women about 'nutrition, domestic hygiene, and health', the colonialism of health care continued with trained nurses who supplanted native health practices. McPherson described nursing as a 'technology of power' that helped white settlers 'remain' where fear of disease may have induced them to leave, and also helped transform the First Nations' cultures by introducing modern medical procedures and practices without regard to previous practices.[74]

Nursing, as a predominantly white profession, was also part of a culture of power with regard to race. In the 1950s the Canadian Nurses' Association (CNA) adopted a formal anti-discrimination policy to combat discrimination against racial minorities in nursing training. Yet as historian Karen Flynn has documented, this policy did not improve the opportunities for nurses emigrating from the Caribbean. During the post-war shortage of nurses, Canadian immigration regulations were relaxed. Flynn has demonstrated that although the Caribbean nurses had better training than European refugee nurses, the Europeans were favoured as immigrants over the Caribbean applicants.[75] McPherson has documented a similar attitude towards First Nation applicants to nursing training schools.[76] Nursing in Canada faced its own struggles to meet community health needs and incorporate a changing population into its health-care provision.

Midwifery also experienced struggles with its identity, as the end of the nineteenth and beginning of the twentieth century heralded restrictions for midwifery practice and increasing assimilation into nursing. Midwives in Quebec, where the earlier French model still influenced maternity care, had initially been supported by local physicians. Official recognition and legal status was granted by the Medical Act of 1788, which also required midwives to attend a six-month training programme in a university.[77] However, according to Laforce, the beginning of an organized resistance to midwifery practice among the medical community came from the Corporation of Doctors. This organization of physicians in Quebec, founded in 1847, controlled hospital training programmes, licensure and regulations for practice for midwives. Although the Corporation was not able to replace midwifery (lay or trained) with obstetrical providers, they were able to institute regulations about the supervision of midwife practice and to control access to training programmes in Quebec. In co-ordination with the new nurse training programmes, midwifery education was moved into nursing departments and eventually subsumed into public health nursing care. By 1944 midwifery certificates were repealed in the province and the only midwives left practicing with official sanction were those in the most remote communities.[78]

This pattern of midwifery care in remote areas for underserved populations played out in other regions of Canada as well. Kate Plummer describes how midwives in Newfoundland practiced alongside medical providers in rural communities with the support of the territorial government. The Act Respecting the Practice of Midwifery passed in 1920 allowed for certification of foreign-trained midwives as well as for lay midwives after completing a three-month training programme.[79] This law remained in place after Newfoundland and Labrador became a province in 1949, but the midwife training programmes died off and the province stopped issuing midwife licenses in 1960. Similarly in Alberta district nurses stationed in remote outposts were trained in midwifery, though never given the actual title of midwife.[80] Judith Zelmanovits has also explored the experiences of nurses stationed in northern outposts, who were expected to provide some level of maternity care, including midwifery, whether or not they were trained for that work.[81] In each of these examples, foreign-trained midwives and nurses played an important role. Plummer notes that the Alberta training midwifery skills programme for district nurses used a Scottish-trained midwife, and a similar programme for outpost nurses at Dalhousie University in Halifax, Nova Scotia, was run by a midwife who received her training at the Frontier school in Kentucky.[82] Zelmanovits notes that the DNHW preferred to hire foreign-trained nurses whose training included practical midwifery.[83] Thus, foreign-trained midwives helped keep alive the practice and profession of midwifery in the years between the Second World War and the 1990s.

Midwifery in Canada disappeared from view for urban and middle-class Canadians through attrition and by the suppression by medical and nursing providers. The advent of the Canadian National Health Service (CNHS) in 1957 further restricted midwifery practice. The Hospital Insurance and Diagnostic Services Act did not outlaw midwifery, but rather simply ignored it, leaving midwives in a professional limbo. Midwifery of all types was not considered an independent profession, rather, at best, it was considered a branch of nursing, and, at worst, an infringement on medical obstetrics. As the Canadian NHS evolved, midwifery was left behind. Canadian midwifery for the most part evaded outright legislation against its practice, but practice was seriously restricted. As midwives did not have hospital privileges and could not bill insurance companies for their services, they were effectively excluded from hospital-based practice, and limited to self-paying clients seeking home births.

However, although the existence of Canadian midwifery was seriously challenged in the twentieth century, Mitchinson has demonstrated that it moved to the margins rather than disappearing entirely.[84] Laura Biggs, historian of Canadian midwifery, suggests that its decline was 'uneven' rather than uniform because of regional cultural, political and market differences.[85] Underpinned by strong community foundations and tacit government approval (or at least governmental neglect), midwifery continued in the form of foreign-trained midwives and nurses who practiced outside the parameters of formal medical care from the mid-twentieth century until the first *official* recognition of the profession in the 1990s in Ontario.[86]

After decades of medicalized birth and midwifery practice limited solely to home birth, in the 1980s midwifery advocates and childbearing consumers began to work together to get trained midwifery recognized by the Canadian NHS.[87] Unlike similar movements in Australia and the United States, the advocacy for midwifery in Canada united direct-entry midwives and nurse-midwives.[88] Ontario was the first Canadian Province to legalize trained midwifery in 1991. The Ontario legislation provided for both direct-entry and nurse-midwifery approaches to midwifery practice, due to the work of midwifery supporters as well as careful study of the various trained midwifery models throughout the world. Today midwifery is an independent profession in Canada, along the lines of midwifery in Britain, and all the provinces of Canada have legalized trained midwifery practice, or have plans to do so.

Comparing National Approaches to Nursing and Midwifery

In 1922, when considering the kinds of nursing schools needed to reconstruct the war-ravaged health infrastructures of Eastern and Southern Europe, the American Elizabeth Crowell commented upon what she believed to be the distinct differences between the educational philosophy and practices of nursing in the United States and United Kingdom. Crowell had been named as a consultant to the Rockefeller Foundation's International Health Board and had travelled extensively throughout England and Europe surveying conditions and recommending particular people and places that would shape the direction of professional nursing on the Continent. Nursing schools in the United States, she believed, were too caught up in the web of a professionalizing agenda to provide a model of the kinds of intensive and personalized care that hospitalized patients on the Continent needed. On the other hand, she continued, the rigorous emphasis on higher education and close supervision in the United States translated perfectly to a robust public health nursing model that would broaden the scope and the practice of the science of public health in both urban and rural areas throughout Europe. Nursing schools in the United Kingdom, by contrast, concentrated on the needs of patients and seemed to graduate nurses with the flexibility to meet the wide-ranging health-care issues that would present in their day-to-day practice within their own particular communities.

While Crowell never directly mentioned midwifery, her comments reflect an appreciation among contemporaries that the United Kingdom and the United States had two distinct approaches to nursing education and practice. Crowell, although American-trained and understanding that she was taking a very controversial position, preferred the British approach: it instilled both the 'spirit of service and the conception of the fundamental, therapeutic value of hygiene, diet and comfort'.[89] As importantly, its flexibility allowed for more than just trained nurses to engage in health work; and Crowell remained impressed with the possibility of other roles for women including that of 'health visitors' teaching well families in their communities the basic tenets of good hygiene, diet, and comfort in ways that reflected the different customs and details of their lives. Crowell lost her campaign to send Continental nurses to the United Kingdom for further training as American nursing leaders quickly intervened with the Foundation to successfully press their vision of education and practice.[90] Those nurses chosen by the Foundation eventually studied nursing education at Teachers College in New York City, nursing practice at the University of Toronto and rural public health practice at Vanderbilt University in Tennessee.

This story illustrates several facets of the nursing and midwifery interface as it moves onto a more international stage. Certainly states, be they local governments or national bodies, had a compelling interest in promoting safe motherhood and healthy citizens. Indicators of maternal and infant mortality were a direct measure of the effectiveness of a public health system charged with the control of infectious and endemic diseases, the safety of health practices, the cleanliness of water and food supplies, and the development of a healthy new generation of men and women. States also less directly controlled nursing and midwifery through policies about who could officially sign birth certificates. Midwifery survived in United Kingdom because of the state's interest in legitimating and regulating its practices. But other states, such as those in Australia who promised higher payments to mothers if they sought a physician rather than a midwife as their birth attendant, linked medicine and nursing, rather than midwifery, more tightly to its programme of white population building. Still others, such as those with large populations of First Nation mothers in Canada or African-American mothers in the United States, seemed indifferent. In these instances, midwifery survived with the tacit complicity of the state and the professions as a way to serve marginalized and underserved populations.

But overlaying the imperatives of states was a broad array of other actors and forces. Some of these are well known and studied. The Rockefeller Foundation, for example, had a strong commitment to partnering with countries across the globe to build their public health infrastructure. Yet this was a particular kind of infrastructure premised on the value of the laboratory, led by physicians trained in the science of public health, and implemented by nurses committed to this vision. And physicians, in another example, had as strong a commitment to safe motherhood and healthy citizens. Yet their vision, coterminous with the development of obstetricians and paediatricians as medical specialists, medicalized pregnancy and childbirth even as it promised pain relief and safety in the wards of hospitals. Both foundations and physicians were relatively hostile to indigenous providers such as midwives.

The role of professional nurses in shaping midwifery practice, however, has been less well studied. Yet, as this chapter has shown, it was not coincidental that the rise in the status and the place of professional nursing was directly and actively linked to the fall in the status and place of midwifery practice in the countries discussed. Indeed, the stronger the emphasis on the professionalizing project, the less likely the practice of lay or trained midwives. This was most apparent in the United States where, throughout the twentieth century, only a very small number of specially trained nurse-midwives survived to serve the poor in mountainous Kentucky or southwestern New Mexico. And yet, even then, the practices were a stop-gap measure to get birthing women to where they themselves wanted to go:

a hospital.[91] In those colonies across the globe where the American emphasis was most strongly felt – the Philippines, Puerto Rico and the Hawaiian Islands – the medicalized model of physician-attended hospital births took hold with nurses themselves leading the vanguard of this movement for safe motherhood.

In those countries that fell within the British sphere of influence – Australia, and parts of Canada in particular – the nursing–midwifery interface was more porous and fell within a tradition of greater inclusivity of other kinds of health-care providers including direct-entry trained midwives and nurse-midwives. Yet, broad national traditions could not compete with local norms, needs, traditions and resources. Despite the universality of childbirth and globally shared twentieth-century experiences of declining birth rates, rising medical authority and economic crises, white middle-class mothers' own intimate and private experiences and expectations determined if there would be a space for midwifery practices to flourish.

But what kinds of midwifery practices? As we look to the twenty-first century new tensions in the nursing–midwifery interface emerge and old ones resurface. In some areas across the globe, nurse-midwives are perceived as part of the medical model that birthing women seek to avoid. In other areas traditional midwives are seen as lacking access to the material and educational resources necessary for safe practices. If we are to ensure that all women are attended by a trained birth attendant as we seek to meet one of the critical United Nations Millennium Development Goals, we must think more systematically about the nursing–midwifery interface – and the new forms it might take in both developed and developing countries.[92]

Notes

1. S. Berger, 'Comparative History', in S. Berger, H. Feldner and K Passmore (eds), *Writing History: Theory and Practice* (London: Arnold, 2003) p. 165.
2. A. Summers, 'A Different Start: Midwifery in South Australia, 1836–1920', *International History of Nursing Journal*, 5:3 (2000) p. 51.
3. R.A. Davies, *'She Did What She Could': A History of the Regulation of Midwifery Practice in Queensland, 1859–1912* (Brisbane: Queensland University of Technology, Center for Health Research, School of Nursing, 2003) p. 111.
4. L. Barclay, 'A Feminist History of Australian Midwifery from Colonization until the 1980s', *Women and Birth*, 21:1 (2008) p. 4.

5. M. Grehan, 'Heroes or Villains? Midwives, Nurses, and Maternity Care in Mid-Nineteenth Century Australia, Free Online Library', 1 January 2009, http://www.thefreelibrary.com/Heroes+or+villains% 3F+Midwives,+nurses,+and+maternity+care+in ... -a0214458324.

6. J. Godden, *Lucy Osburn, A Lady Displaced: Florence Nightingale's Envoy to Australia* (Sydney: Sydney University Press, 2006) p. 84.

7. J. Barber, 'All the Young Men Gone: Losing Men in the Gentrification of Australian Nursing, *c.*1860–1899', *Nursing Inquiry*, 3:4 (1996) 218–24; J. Godden, 'Hospitals', *Sydney Journal*, 1:2 (16 June 2008) pp. 1–10.

8. This paper will not address the history of aboriginal birth practices or midwifery due to a lack of secondary resources available on the subject.

9. Summers, 'A Different Start', p. 52.

10. M. Grehan, 'Gillbee, Sarah Ann: Biographical Entry – Royal Women's Hospital History', 26 November 2006, http://www.thewomenshistory. org.au/biogs/e000068b.htm; Grehan, 'Heroes or villains?'

11. Barclay, 'Feminist History', p. 5; Summers, 'Different Start', p. 53.

12. N. Purcal, 'The Politics of Midwifery Education and Training in New South Wales during the Last Decades of the Nineteenth Century', *Women and Birth*, 21:1 (2008) pp. 21–5; F. Bogossian, 'A Review of Midwifery Legislation in Australia: History, Current State and Future Directions', *Australian College of Midwives Incorporated Journal* (March 1998) p. 24.

13. Fahy, 'An Australian History of the Subordination of Midwifery', *Women and Birth*, 20:1 (2007) p. 27.

14. Fahy, 'Australian History', pp. 27–8.

15. Fahy, 'Australian History', p. 28.

16. Summers, 'A Different Start', p. 55.

17. Godden, *Lucy Osburn*.

18. J. Godden, 'Bathsheba Ghost, Matron of the Sydney Infirmary 1852–66: A Silenced Life', *Labour History*, no. 87 (1 November 2004) p. 55.

19. J. Godden and S. Forsyth, 'Defining Relationships and Limiting Power: Two Leaders of Australian Nursing, 1868–1904', *Nursing Inquiry*, 7:1 (2000) 10–19.

20. Barber, 'All the Young Men Gone'.

21. S.B. McGahey, 'Nursing Organization in Australia', *The American Journal of Nursing*, 1:3 (1900) 237.

22. H. Witham, 'ANF Celebrates 75 Years', *Australian Nurses' Journal*, 6:8 (1999) 15.

23. Witham, 'ANF'; Australian Nursing and Midwifery Accreditation Council, 'Registered Nurse and Midwife Education in Australia' (February 2008), http://www.anmc.org.au/userfiles/file/guidelines_ and_position_statements/Registered%20Nurse%20and%20Midwife %20Education%20in%20Australia.pdf.

24. Barclay, 'Feminist History', p. 6.
25. A. Summers, 'The Lost Voice of Midwifery: Midwives, Nurses and the Nurses Registration Act of South Australia', *Collegian: Journal of the Royal College of Nursing Australia*, 5:3 (1998) 18.
26. Bogossian, 'Review', p. 25.
27. Bogossian, 'Review'.
28. Godden, Lucy Osburn, p. 200.
29. Barclay, 'Feminist History', p. 5.
30. Summers, 'Lost Voice', p. 19.
31. Summers, 'Lost Voice', p. 21.
32. Bogossian, 'Review'.
33. P. Glover, 'Australia Makes History: The First Three-Year Bachelor of Midwifery Course of Studies: Pauline Glover', Associate Professor of Midwifery & Nursing, Flinders University, Adelaide, describes a pioneering addition to midwifery education in Australia, 2005, http://findarticles.com/p/articles/mi_m0KTL/is_2_18/ai_n17209364/.
34. H. James and E. Willis, 'The Professionalization of Midwifery through Education or Politics?' *The Australian Journal of Midwifery*, 14:4 (2001) 27–30.
35. L. Mckenna and C. Rolls, 'Bachelor of Midwifery: Reflections on the First 5 Years from Two Victorian Universities', *Women and Birth*, 20:2 (2007) 81–4.
36. 'Table Bd241–256 – Physicians, Dentists, Nurses, and Medical, Dental, and Nursing Schools and Students: 1810–1995', *Historical Statistics of the United States Millennial Edition Online*, 1 July 2010, http://proxy.library.upenn.edu:5403/HSUSWeb/search/searchTable.do?id= Bd241-256; P. D'Antonio, *American Nursing: A History of Knowledge, Authority, and the Meaning of Work* (Baltimore: Johns Hopkins University Press, 2010) p. 26.
37. D'Antonio, *American Nursing*, pp. 51–3.
38. D'Antonio, *American Nursing*, pp. 1–26.
39. K. Buhler-Wilkerson, *False Dawn: The Rise and Fall of Public Health Nursing in America* (New York: Garland Publishing, 1983) p. 98.
40. Buhler-Wilkerson, *No Place Like Home: A History of Nursing and Home Care in the United States* (Baltimore: John Hopkins University Press, 2001) p. 63.
41. J.L. Koslow, *Cultivating Health: Los Angeles Women and Public Health Reform* (New Brunswick: Rutgers University Press, 2009); A.L. Fairchild et al., *Searching Eyes: Privacy, the State, and Disease Surveillance in America* (Berkeley: University of California Press, 2007); A.M. Kraut, *Silent Travelers: Germs, Genes, and the Immigrant Menace* (Baltimore: Johns Hopkins University Press, 1995); George Rosen, *A History of Public Health* (Baltimore: Johns Hopkins University Press, 1993).

42. K. Buhler-Wilkerson, *False Dawn;* G.J. Fraser, *African American Midwifery in the South: Dialogues of Birth, Race, and Memory*, 1st edn (Cambridge, MA: Harvard University Press, 1998); J.P. Brickman, 'Public Health, Midwives, and Nurses, 1880–1930', in E. C. Lagemann (ed.), *Nursing History; New Perspectives, New Possibilities* (New York: Teachers College Press, 1983) 35–88; F. Kobrin, 'The American Midwife Controversy: A Crisis in Professionalism', *Bulletin of the History of Medicine*, 40 (1966) pp. 350–63.

43. L.T. Ulrich, *A Midwife's Tale: The Life of Martha Ballard, Based on Her Diary 1785–1812* (New York: Alfred A. Knopf, 1990) p. 162.

44. S.L. Smith, *Japanese American Midwives; Culture, Community, and Health Politics, 1880–1950* (Chicago: University of Illinois Press, 2005); C. Borst, *Catching Babies: The Professionalization of Childbirth, 1870–1920* (Cambridge, MA: Harvard University Press, 1995); J.W. Leavitt, *Brought to Bed: Childbearing in America, 1750 to 1950* (New York: Oxford University Press, 1986).

45. Smith, *Japanese American Midwives*; L.A. Walsh, 'Midwives as Wives and Mothers: Urban Midwives in the Early Twentieth Century', *Nursing History Review*, 2 (1994) 51–65.

46. S. Smith, 'White Nurses, Black Midwives, and Public Health in Mississippi, 1920–1950', in J.W. Leavitt (ed.), *Women and Health in America: Historical Readings* (Madison, WI: University of Wisconsin Press, 1984) pp. 448–58; N. Devitt, 'The Statistical Case for the Elimination of the Midwife: Fact versus Prejudice, 1890–1930', in Leavitt (ed.), *Women and Health in America*, pp. 169–86; I. Loudon, 'Midwives and the Quality of Maternal Care', in H. Marland and A.M. Rafferty (eds), *Midwives, Society, and Childbirth: Debates and Controversies in the Modern Period* (London/New York: Routledge, 1997) pp. 180–200.

47. Z.O. Jones, 'Knowledge Systems in Conflict: The Regulation of African American Midwifery', *Nursing History Review*, 12 (2004) 167–84.

48. K. Dawley, 'Ideology and Self-Interest: Nursing, Medicine, and the Elimination of the Midwife', *Nursing History Review*, 9 (2001) 99–126.

49. Leavitt, *Brought to Bed*.

50. K.L. Dawley, 'Leaving the Nest: Nurse-Midwifery in the United States 1940–1980' (PhD Dissertation, University of Pennsylvania, 2001) pp. 142–8.

51. L.E. Ettinger, *Nurse-Midwifery: The Birth of a New American Profession* (Columbus, OH: Ohio State University Press, 2006).

52. M. Breckinridge, *Wide Neighborhoods, a Story of the Frontier Nursing Service* (New York: Harper, 1952) pp. 93–100.

53. M.B. Goan, *Mary Breckinridge: The Frontier Nursing Service and Rural Health in Appalachia* (Chapel Hill, NC: University of North Carolina Press, 2008).

54. A.Z. Cockerham and A.W. Keeling, 'Finance and Faith at the Catholic Maternity Institute, Santa Fe, New Mexico, 1944 1969', *Nursing History Review*, 18 (2010) pp. 151–66.
55. K. Dawley, 'American Nurse-Midwifery: A Hyphenated Profession with a Conflicted Identity', *Nursing History Review*, 13 (2005) p. 152.
56. Dawley, 'American Nurse-Midwifery', p. 152.
57. Dawley, 'American Nurse-Midwifery', p. 148.
58. Dawley, 'American Nurse-Midwifery', p. 154.
59. V. Strong-Boag, 'Making a Difference: The History of Canada's Nurses', *Canadian Bulletin of Medical History/Bulletin canadien d'histoire de la médecine*, 8:2 (1991) p. 240.
60. Strong-Boag, 'Making a Difference', p. 240.
61. Strong-Boag, 'Making a Difference', p. 240.
62. H. Laforce, 'The Different Stages of the Elimination of Midwives in Quebec', in E. Van Teijlingen et al. (eds), *Midwifery and the Medicalization of Childbirth: Comparative Perspectives* (Commack, NJ: Nova Science Publishers, 2000) p. 118
63. L.Biggs, 'Rethinking the History of Midwifery in Canada', in I.L. Bourgeault, C. Benoit and R. Davis-Floyd (eds), *Reconceiving Midwifery* (Montréal: McGill-Queen's University Press, 2004) p. 30.
64. W. Mitchinson, *Giving Birth in Canada, 1900–1950* (Toronto: University of Toronto Press, 2002) p. 79.
65. Biggs, 'Rethinking'; N. Langford, 'Childbirth on the Canadian Prairies, 1880–1930', in C.A. Cavanaugh and R.R. Warne (eds), *Telling Tales: Essays in Western Women's History* (Vancouver, BC: UBC Press, 2000) pp. 147–73.
66. D. Dodd, 'Helen MacMurchy: Popular Midwifery and Maternity Services for Canadian Pioneer Women', in D.E. Dodd and D. Gorham (eds), *Caring and Curing: Historical Perspectives on Women and Healing in Canada* (Ottawa: University of Ottawa Press, 1994) pp. 135–62.
67. K. Plummer, 'From Nursing Outposts to Contemporary Midwifery in 20th Century Canada', *Journal of Midwifery & Women's Health*, 45:2 (2000) 169–75.
68. J.M. Gibbon and M.S. Mathewson, *Three Centuries of Canadian Nursing* (Toronto: Macmillan Co of Canada, 1947).
69. S.M. Reverby, *Ordered to Care: The Dilemma of American Nursing, 1850–1945* (Cambridge: Cambridge University Press, 1987) p. 80.
70. Strong-Boag, 'Making a Difference', p. 236.
71. Langford, 'Childbirth', p. 148.
72. Laforce, 'Different Stages', p. 123.
73. K. McPherson, 'Nursing and Colonization: The Work of Indian Health Service Nurses in Manitoba', in G. Feldberg et al. (eds), *Women, Health and Nation: Canada and the United States since 1945* (Montréal: McGill-Queen's University Press, 2003) pp. 223–46.

74. McPherson, 'Nursing', pp. 225–27.
75. K. Flynn, 'Race, the State, and Caribbean Immigrant Nurses, 1950–1962', in Feldberg et al. (eds), *Women*, pp. 247–63.
76. McPherson, 'Nursing', pp. 225–27, 235.
77. Plummer, 'From Nursing Outposts', p. 169.
78. Laforce, 'Different Stages'; 'A Summary of the History of Midwifery in Canada', n.d., http://www.ucs.mun.ca/~pherbert/Historyofmidincanada.html.
79. Plummer, 'From Nursing Outposts', p. 170.
80. Plummer, 'From Nursing Outposts', p. 170.
81. J.B. Zelmanovits, ' "Midwife Preferred": Maternity Care in Outpost Nursing Stations in Northern Canada', in Feldberg et al. (eds), *Women*, p. 173.
82. Plummer, 'From Nursing Outposts', pp. 171, 173.
83. Zelmanovits, 'Midwife Preferred', p. 166.
84. Mitchinson, *Giving Birth*.
85. Biggs, 'Rethinking', p. 30.
86. Plummer, 'From Nursing Outposts'.
87. I.L. Bourgeault and M. Fynes, 'Integration Lay and Nurse-Midwifery into the U.S. and Canadian Health Care Systems', *Social Science & Medicine*, 44:7 (1997) p. 1058.
88. Bourgeault and Fynes, 'Integration'.
89. Rockefeller Archives Center, RF, RG 1.1, Series 700, Box 19, Folder 137F, Elizabeth Crowell to George Vincent, 27 August 1922.
90. J. Farley, *To Cast Out Disease: A History of the International Health Division of the Rockefeller Foundation, 1913–1951* (Oxford: Oxford University Press, 2004) pp. 28–9.
91. Cockerham and Keeling, 'Finance'; Leavitt, *Brought to Bed*.
92. 'United Nations Millennium Development Goals', n.d., http://www.un.org/millenniumgoals/maternal.shtml.

9

Nursing and Midwifery: An Uneasy Alliance or Natural Bedfellows?

Billie Hunter and Anne Borsay

The relationship between nursing and midwifery is the subject of contemporary debate and opinion, often heated and polarized.[1] As Rosemary Mander has wryly observed, it is a relationship 'which has a tendency to generate more heat than light'.[2] Midwives hold dear to the notion of being 'different' to nursing, claiming a unique role and identity which are experienced as in danger of being subsumed into nursing.[3] Nurses, on the other hand, may view midwifery as part and parcel of the nursing profession. Indeed, some argue that clinging to notions of separateness only serves to dilute common goals, and that development of both professions would benefit from incorporating midwifery as a specialism within a family of generic nursing interests.

The nature of the relationship between nursing and midwifery differs internationally. In some countries, the two professions have evolved separately (e.g. in the Netherlands and Denmark), while in others it is possible to practise midwifery only as a nurse-midwife (e.g. in Sweden and some parts of the United States). There is an apparent trend towards establishing direct-entry programmes in the United Kingdom, Canada and Australia, although the rationale for this may differ between countries. It is claimed that 'nearly one half of the world's midwives are also nurses'.[4] Dual-qualified practitioners are particularly common in the developing world and in remote areas,[5] where it may be more appropriate to employ multi-skilled practitioners able to meet the diverse health needs of whole communities. It is therefore seen as imperative for nurses and midwives to work together as 'truly respected partners and collaborators with many others based on a common goal of healthy people'.[6] However, this argument does appear to gloss over the historical evidence of the professional rivalries which have certainly existed across the world. For example, in early accounts of the International Midwives Union (now the International Confederation of Midwives) concern is expressed about the encroachment of nurses, especially district nurses and maternity nurses, into what was seen as midwifery territory: working with women and their families in the community.[7]

In the United Kingdom, the two professions have evolved to exist side by side. Since 1979 they have been regulated by the same body (initially, the United Kingdom Central Council for Nursing, Midwifery and Health Visiting (UKCC), and currently the Nursing and Midwifery Council (NMC)), but they are represented by different Royal Colleges. They share some professional regulations and standards (e.g. the *NMC Code: Standards of Conduct, Performance and Ethics for Nurses and Midwives*), but midwifery also has a number of midwifery-specific rules and directives (i.e. the *NMC Midwives Rules and Standards*). Likewise, there is some overlap in clinical skills (e.g. monitoring vital signs, giving injections), but many skills are unique to each profession. It is not necessary to have a nursing qualification to train as a midwife, or vice versa, and increasingly in the United Kingdom, midwives are likely to have sole rather than dual qualifications. However, numbers of nurses far exceed those of midwives (494,020 nurses to 33,305 midwives in 2007–08).[8] As a result, it has been common practice for 'the larger body to rationalize absorption of the smaller',[9] with nurses representing both professions at a senior level. For example, all four UK countries have a Chief Nurse, who represents all nurses and midwives and may or may not have a midwifery qualification; in most UK Universities, it is common for nursing and midwifery to be located in the same faculty, if not the same School or Department.

In order to better understand the nuances of this complex interprofessional relationship, it is necessary to consider the respective histories of nursing and midwifery. The previous chapters have described the different historical backgrounds of the two professions, providing evidence that it was not until relatively recently, in the later years of the nineteenth century, that there was any significant convergence. This chapter provides a comparative analysis of these histories, focusing on UK health care to explore the synergies and tensions which have emerged over the past three centuries. It is notable that, despite anecdotal evidence of the tensions which exist between nursing and midwifery, there is little critical analysis evident in the professional or academic literature. To do justice to the complexity of the topic would require greater in-depth enquiry than is possible here. However, it is hoped that this chapter will stimulate debate and begin to address this gap in our understanding.

The chapter begins with a consideration of nursing and midwifery prior to their respective Registration Acts, before discussing the effects of registration and professionalization. A number of key similarities are noted: the focus on providing direct client/patient care; the gendered nature of the work; and the twentieth-century move towards establishing graduate-level qualifications and an underpinning research base. There are, however, a number of areas where the two professions diverge: for example, in the specificity or generality of their roles; in the extent of their occupational autonomy and the nature of their professional boundaries; in their respective relationships with medical practitioners; and in the influence of the United States on professionalization strategies.

Before the Registration Acts: Parallel Roles

In the eighteenth and early nineteenth centuries, the roles of midwife and nurse appear to have been undertaken by different groups of women, whose activities were marked more by difference than similarity. Nursing had its background in providing hands-on care for the sick and in supplying domestic care in institutions such as workhouses and asylums, as well as within religious orders. Both activities were seen as an extension of women's role in the home. As Anne Borsay and Christine Hallett describe in Chapters 2 and 3, domestic care included housekeeping, ordering supplies, cleaning, keeping patients fed and clean, and giving treatments. Any type of training for this role was rare until the mid-1850s.

In contrast, in Chapters 5 and 6 Helen King and Alison Nuttall describe how midwives focused specifically on attending women in childbirth, and thus needed to acquire a particular set of skills, over and above the caring qualities attributed to being a woman. They provide evidence that midwifery training, either by apprenticeship or formal instruction, began before nursing training. Apart from lying-in hospitals, the locus of midwifery care tended to be outside institutions until long after the 1902 Midwives' Act, with community-based midwives attending women in their own homes. This meant that midwives were unlikely to be engaged in the domestic duties which were part of the nurses' role. However, once midwifery began to move into hospitals in the 1930s and 1940s, and it became more common for midwives to have undertaken previous nurse training, ward cleaning and other 'housework'-related tasks feature more heavily in the accounts of midwifery work.[10]

This community-based locus of care also meant that, in comparison with nurses, midwives were able to practise autonomously rather than working under surveillance. As a result, midwives were often in direct competition with men–midwives and doctors. Although the focus of the midwife's work was usually on 'normal cases', with doctors being called for assistance should major difficulties arise, there were those who proposed that midwives should extend their role to become the providers of all maternity care, that is, for both normal and abnormal cases. One of these protagonists was Florence Nightingale, more commonly associated with nursing than midwifery. She made an interesting distinction between the extended length of training she considered ideal for a midwife, and that which would be sufficient to qualify as a maternity nurse:

> I call a midwife a woman who has received such a training, scientific and practical, as that she can undertake *all cases* of parturition, normal and abnormal, subject only to consultation, like any other accoucher. Such training could not be given in less than two years. . . . no training of six months could enable a woman to be more than a Midwifery Nurse.[11]

The respective relationships of nurses and midwives with doctors also differed, with nurses unlikely to be in competition with doctors. As medical knowledge and practice began to evolve in the early nineteenth century, doctors needed the assistance of additional staff with sufficient skills and clinical knowledge to follow their treatment instructions and report any changes in the patient's condition. These assistants were clearly in a support role, and needed to be willing to obey the doctor's directions and follow these to the letter. As the nineteenth century progressed, nurses increasingly took on this role, although how much this was a considered decision on behalf of nursing leaders, and how much it was a co-evolution of the two roles is unclear. In contrast, there was much less expectation that midwives would function as the doctor's assistant, although this increasingly became the case during the twentieth century.

Campaigns for Registration: Courting and Rebuffs

The late nineteenth-century campaigns for nursing and midwifery registration reveal emerging links between the two occupations, and the appearance of a new breed of practitioner, qualified as both nurse and midwife. It is noteworthy that midwives such as Rosalind Paget and Zepherina Veitch, who led the movement for midwifery registration, were also nurses. Nursing and midwifery campaigners were usually socially well-connected women of independent means and philanthropic backgrounds. They saw the opportunity for carving out new professional occupations for educated, middle-class women, in keeping with the emerging interest in active citizenship for women and the revived movement for women's suffrage.[12] These new professional roles were also congruent with the perceived urgent need to improve the welfare of working-class families. Both midwife and nurse were exhorted to take on the role of 'Health Missioner', 'making herself a little centre of light and knowledge amidst the ignorance and misery she longs to mitigate'.[13]

However, the aims of nursing and midwifery leaders were not always congruent and there is evidence of competing goals and claims for legitimacy. The most often cited of these tensions is the clash between Ethel Bedford Fenwick, founder of the British Nurses' Association in 1887, and Rosalind Paget, leader of the Midwives' Institute (founded in 1881 as the Matrons' Aid Society or Trained Midwives' Registration Society).[14] Bedford Fenwick had sought the support of the Midwives' Institute in her campaign for nurses' registration, apparently hoping that the backing of the longer established midwives' organization would help her to fast track the process of nurse registration. Although she did succeed in gaining support from some educated nurse-midwives with the enticement of a higher-level grade for midwives on her proposed BNA register, the majority of Midwives' Institute members were 'not seduced and Mrs Fenwick's overtures [were] met with a rebuff'.[15] Mander suggests that this was because the midwifery leaders' energies were needed for their own registration and legislation struggles. These were gathering momentum but meeting resistance from doctors, who wrongly blamed midwives for high levels of maternal and neonatal mortality.[16] It is also likely that midwifery leaders were not convinced that there was substantial common ground between the two campaigns. In a letter to the *Nursing Record* (of which Bedford Fenwick was editor), Jane Wilson, an active Midwives' Institute member, wrote that 'midwives, unlike nurses, were independent practitioners in their own right, with sole responsibility for their patients. Their registration was therefore a more urgent matter and should be dealt with separately.'[17]

As a result of being 'spurned',[18] Bedford Fenwick led a vigorous campaign against midwifery regulation. In an article in the *Nursing Record*, she accused midwives of being 'an anachronism' and an 'historical curiosity'.[19] Her various attempts to gain midwives' support for a joint register failed, indicating that Bedford Fenwick lacked insight into how midwives saw their role and purpose as being fundamentally different to that of nurses. For example, the large meeting which she convened at the Mansion House in London, in an attempt to garner the support of obstetricians, backfired when one eminent obstetrician, Dr Matthews Duncan, outraged Midwives' Institute members by stating that midwives and midwifery nurses were the same thing.[20] This lack of understanding confirmed the Midwives' Institute members' view of the inappropriateness of the BNA's mission, and consolidated their commitment to going it alone, a strategy which was to prove successful with the passing of the Midwives' Act in 1902.

Despite these conflicts, towards the end of the nineteenth century there is evidence of developing links between the two professions. For example, early midwifery training programmes (LOS), such as that offered by the London Obstetrical Society, were of reduced length for those already in possession of a nursing qualification. The 1902 Midwives' Act introduced compulsory three-month training for midwives, which was increased in 1916 to six months, with a two-month reduction for qualified trained nurses.[21] Reduced length of midwifery training for qualified nurses remains the case in twenty-first century UK midwifery education, where a midwifery qualification can be gained in 18 months if a nursing qualification is held, as opposed to 3 years.

Despite the early and equally passionate campaigning for nursing registration by many nursing leaders, this took much longer to achieve, with the Nurses Registration Act not being passed until 1919. The reasons for this difference are multi-faceted. Certainly the campaign for nurse registration was significantly delayed by the First World War, but this does not fully explain the difference. It is probably significant that the campaign for nursing registration was bedevilled by infighting between nurses. Indeed, as Christine Hallett describes in Chapter 3, some of the most vociferous opponents to nurses' registration were nurses themselves. This was not the case in midwifery, where most midwives appear to support registration, even if the preferred form that this might take differed.[22] Midwives' key opponents were the medical profession, many of whom feared the competition for business that a new breed of trained midwives might present. Thus the midwifery campaign was characterized by a relatively unified response to the challenge from their medical rivals, while the nursing campaign was distinguished by its lack of internal consensus.

After the Registration Acts: Growing Allegiance

Once both nursing and midwifery registration had been achieved, there is evidence that the two 'new' professions increasingly began to share common concerns. Although the specific role of the midwife was enshrined in statute, and direct-entry training remained (albeit with a rather tenuous foothold at times), it became increasingly common for midwives to be dual-qualified in the first part of the twentieth century. Indeed, 'doing your midders' became something that nurses routinely undertook after qualifying, whether or not they intended to practice. This trend was acknowledged in a change to midwifery education in 1938, which divided the course into two parts: Part One was hospital-based and Part Two was community-based.[23] It was possible to practise as a midwife only if both parts had been completed. Many nurses undertook Part One only: while this meant they were unable to practise midwifery, it may have provided insights into the work of the midwife (albeit within the hospital) which in turn may have helped to break down professional boundaries.

It is difficult to know how much midwives and nurses encouraged, resisted or were neutral to this blurring of professional boundaries. The international midwifery community continued to make a clear demarcation between the two professions, stating that the work of the nurse was to 'nurse her medical patients and the midwife to look after her patients in confinement and her nurslings'.[24] In Britain, however, it became increasingly common for midwives to be referred to as nurses, even if they were not nurse-trained. For example, describing her visits around the village on her bicycle, district midwife Mary

Wroe recalled: 'all the shopkeepers knew you – "There's the Nurse going along." '[25]

There are other notable semantic ambiguities and evidence of role blurring. For example, the early journal *Nursing Notes* was in fact the official journal of the Midwives' Institute, later re-named the Midwives Chronicle. And in a 1917 report *Physical Welfare of Mothers and Children,* Dr Janet Campbell noted: 'The midwife occupies an exceptional position *in the nursing profession* [our italics] in that she is called upon during her ordinary work to be directly responsible for the lives of two patients, mother and child.'[26] Arguing for the need for more educated women to train as midwives, Campbell notes that as a result 'the old stigma attached to the term midwife will disappear, and the title will revive the respect and recognition which are its due'.[27]

These incongruities appear to suggest that the public status of nurses was higher than midwives, at that period at least. This is surprising given that midwifery regulation was longer established, although it may have been that the more recent campaigning for nurse registration had raised public awareness of the role and skills of the nurse. The public image of nursing had also been raised by the work of Florence Nightingale, who had achieved iconic status in the nation's imagination. Nursing was fast becoming an attractive vocation for 'respectable girls' and as Donnison observes 'was more in tune with current ideas of female propriety than was midwifery'.[28] She notes that the 'new' nurse would be relatively protected, living in the hospital under the gaze of the matron, or caring for patients in well-off families. In contrast, the work of the midwife was 'unmentionable in polite female society, lay usually among the poor, and might bring comparatively little return',[29] an observation which resonates with Janet Campbell's allusion to the 'stigma' of midwifery work. It is also the case that 'new' midwives were keen to distance themselves from handywomen, which adopting the title 'Nurse' might assist. These factors are all likely to have contributed to a diminished status for midwifery.

It is certainly the case that nursing was a larger and hence more influential profession. It is therefore quite likely that some midwifery leaders may have seen an increased alliance with nursing as a means of elevating the image of the profession and increasing legitimation, especially now that nursing registration had been achieved. Certainly this appears to have been the case in many countries where midwifery has attempted to secure professional status. In the United States, for example, De Vries argues that midwives formed an alliance with the established profession of nursing precisely in order to prevent the extinction of midwifery.[30]

1950–2000: Integration and Resistance

During the 1950s and 1960s, when most British midwifery care re-located to hospital settings, it became increasingly difficult to differentiate between the two professions. The upsurge in obstetric medicine and the concurrent shift in attitudes to childbirth and risk, described in Chapter 7, led to an increasing expectation that midwives would function as the doctor's assistant in medically managed childbirth. Someone was needed to monitor the intravenous infusion of syntocinon when labour was induced and to observe the recordings of the electronic foetal heart monitor, as became common practice in the 1960s and 1970s. That someone was the midwife. It is unclear whether midwives initially saw this as an extension of their role or a restriction. Certainly, many midwives were convinced of the benefits offered by scientific medicine.[31] There is little evidence of any concern about the role shift from autonomous practitioner to that of obstetric nurse being voiced until the 1970s.[32]

The integrating trend of the 1950s and 1960s culminated a number of initiatives in the 1970s aimed at further combining the two professions. The proposals for a unified regulatory body and shared pre-registration education set out in the *Briggs Report* of 1972 met with considerable resistance, mainly from some midwives who were once again concerned that their specific needs would be subsumed by nursing. Despite these protests, shared regulation went ahead, with the 1979 Nurses, Midwives and Health Visitors Act establishing the UKCC (with a concession to midwives by the inclusion of a Midwifery Committee).

However, the changes to pre-registration education proposed by the UKCC Project 2000 had a rockier passage. The main initial proposals were for a common foundation programme for all nursing specialities, followed by individual 'branch' programmes.[33] Although the UKCC accepted that 'midwifery is a profession different from, but complementary to nursing',[34] midwifery was named as one of these nursing specialties, alongside mental health nursing and children's nursing. This was met with vehement protest from many midwives:

> Wake up! We must not allow ourselves to be engulfed and swamped by these proposals, which would not produce the midwife practitioners

we need and would, once and for all, see the demise of midwifery as a separate profession.[35]

Ultimately, resistance from midwives meant that this aspect of the proposal was dropped, and Project 2000 went ahead to become established in an amended form for nurses. However, traces of this integrative approach remain to the current day. For example, in many universities, midwifery students on direct-entry programmes undertake placements on nursing wards and share lectures with nursing students. Other Project 2000 recommendations which affected both nurses and midwives were adopted: nursing and midwifery schools moved into Higher Education and were situated in universities, students became additional to the paid workforce and there was a new focus on health rather than illness. The emphasis was on creating 'knowledgeable doers', that is practitioners who had high levels of both theoretical knowledge and practical knowhow.[36] The transition from separate Colleges of Nursing and Colleges of Midwifery situated close to hospitals, to amalgamated Schools located in universities brought benefits and challenges.[37] While conferring 'proper' student status on these undergraduates, educators and clinicians became increasingly concerned about the separation of education and practice, and the resulting potential for a 'theory–practice gap'. These concerns grew, compounded by problems with new graduates who appeared to lack the skills needed to practise. In 1998 the UKCC commissioned a review of nursing and midwifery pre-registration education, to propose 'a way forward for pre-registration education that enabled fitness for practice based on health care need'.[38] The resulting 'Fitness for Practice Report' made a number of recommendations aimed at increasing practice skills, including a competency-based approach, more rigorous practice assessments and a period of supervised clinical practice prior to registration.[39] This initiative is still a 'work in progress'.

Discussion: An Uneasy Alliance or Natural Bedfellows?

The previous historical overview suggests a number of key similarities and differences between nursing and midwifery, which will be summarized and evaluated in this concluding section. Of course, there are many other significant groups of specialist nurses, for example intensive-care nurses, mental health nurses, health visitors, community nurses and advanced nurse practitioners, who have differing role boundaries and levels of responsibility and autonomy. However, this discussion, by necessity, considers nurses as a homogenous group and refers most commonly to the practice of general nurses.

Both nursing and midwifery are female-dominated professions which work alongside medicine, although the nature of their respective relationships with medicine differs, as does the extent of their occupational jurisdiction and the level of autonomy claimed. Both engage in 'people work',[40] addressing individual health needs and providing direct care which entails both emotional and physical labour. Both nurses and midwives cite the importance of 'wanting to make a difference' in their reasons for career choice and accounts of job satisfaction.[41] Midwives have traditionally claimed that their work centres on health and well-being, and that this distinguishes them from nursing, with its disease and illness focus. However, the Project 2000 shift to a 'health' model for nursing education, which also underpins many nursing specialties, means that this is no longer a unique signifier, if indeed it ever truly was.

Both professions have their roots in the craft skills of untrained or apprentice-trained local women, with eighteenth- and nineteenth-century midwives more usually situated in local communities. The campaigns for professionalization occurred more or less concurrently, directed by well-connected, articulate female leaders operating within the context of a broader sea-change in the status and aspirations of nineteenth-century women. These leaders harnessed the support of influential (mainly male) politicians, philanthropists and doctors to spearhead lengthy, but ultimately successful, campaigns for professional regulation and registration during the late nineteenth and early twentieth centuries.

The professional projects of nurses and midwives have employed similar strategies, although there are also important differences. In the second part of the twentieth century, an emphasis on education rather than training was seen as the route for achieving professionalization, and both professions moved the preparation of learners into higher education. There were resultant challenges, both for developing academic credibility with new university colleagues, and for maintaining clinical credibility with practice-based colleagues. Both nursing and midwifery academics were challenged by grass-roots workers regarding the perceived academicization of the profession and fears of a growing theory–practice gap. Concerns about whether graduates are 'fit for practice' persist, particularly in nursing where media stories portray graduate nurses as being 'too clever to care'. Thus, while nurses and midwives may have enhanced their intellectual status in relation to academia, there is still considerable work to do in improving their public image and in convincing the public of the value of creating 'knowledgeable doers'. Interestingly, it is the caring aspect of nurses' public image that appears to need current attention. For midwives, concerns are more related to their relative invisibility and lack of public understanding about their distinctiveness from nursing.[42]

A particular challenge for both professions has been the need to create a research evidence base to underpin practice. For both, this goal remains in its infancy when compared with the well-established evidence base of many other professions and academic disciplines. However, the results of the most recent UK Research Assessment Exercise (RAE) in 2008 showed rapid developments in this area, with the UK Council of Deans of Health commenting on the 'tremendous advances in nursing and midwifery research in the UK since the last RAE in 2001. It now confirms the role of nursing and midwifery as a world class subject area in higher education.'[43]

Nursing made earlier moves than midwifery to establish itself as a research-based profession. Nursing degree programmes were first set up in the 1970s, whereas the first midwifery degree programme was not established until 1989.[44] Similarly, nursing began to develop a body of research-based knowledge earlier than midwifery. The first nursing research reports, such as *The Proper Study of the Nurse*[45] and *Towards a Theory of Nursing*,[46] published in the 1970s, are still viewed as classic papers. The first nursing professors were appointed before midwifery professors: Margaret Scott-Wright was appointed as the first UK Chair of Nursing Studies at Edinburgh University in 1971[47]; Lesley Page was the first UK Professor of Midwifery at Queen Charlotte's College, later known as Thames Valley University, in 1991.[48]

It appears that the influence of the United States was highly significant for these nursing developments. US nursing had a strong influence on the development of UK nursing education and research, evident in the North American theoretical nursing models which dominated UK nursing education in the 1970s and 1980s. The same did not apply to midwifery. The very limited development of midwifery in the United States, described in Chapter 8, meant that US midwifery had little to offer UK midwives – in fact, the influence was in the opposite direction, with British approaches to midwifery being held up as exemplary by many American midwives. There was little attempt to develop mid- or grand-range theories of midwifery practice in the way that nurses had.[49] Midwifery research in the United Kingdom was influenced more by maternity research conducted by social scientists and doctors than by nursing research. For example, the National Perinatal Epidemiology Unit had a significant effect on the work of early midwifery researchers such as Sleep and Renfrew.[50] There was a tendency to focus on clinical care issues such as perineal suturing and breastfeeding, rather than theory building or exploring the nature of midwifery.

A key focus of much nursing research and scholarship in the 1990s, discussed in detail in Chapter 4, was the exploration of 'what is nursing?' The concerns about the nature and scope of nursing practice, which had first been raised in the nineteenth century, remained problematic. Nursing had a divided focus: providing patient care and acting as an assistant to the doctor. Debates raged about whether patient care required a specialized body of knowledge held by registered nurses or could be delegated to a 'second-level' carer, for example the State Enrolled Nurse (who existed until the mid-1990s) or to auxiliary nurses and health-care assistants. The late twentieth century saw academic moves to elevate the value and status of hands-on nursing care, discussed in Chapter 4, although these were frequently at odds with the realities of providing care in an under-staffed and poorly resourced National Health Service (NHS).

By comparison with nursing, the focus of midwifery was – and is – clear. This may have presented both advantages and disadvantages. There were no similar debates about 'what is midwifery', because the very specific, focused nature of midwifery meant that midwives knew what their role was. Historically, midwives have always cared for women and babies during pregnancy, birth and postpartum, thus ensuring clarity of purpose. Even though the UK midwives' role has expanded into public health (screening, health promotion, domestic abuse, child protection), and the scope of the midwives' role may vary globally, its essence and primary focus remain consistent.[51] However, while this clarity of purpose may be seen as conferring advantages on midwives, it may also have led to some unanticipated consequences. It could be argued that midwives' specific focus on women, birth and babies has limited their wider influence, with midwives characterized as a 'single-issue' profession, of relevance only to women at a specific period of their lives. It is also the case that midwives' primary emphasis on women's concerns and being 'with woman' may have led to a de-valuing of the role, particularly in cultures where women are not valued and the equal rights of women are not recognized.

By contrast, nurses may care for anyone in a community at times of ill-health: old or young, male or female, high or low status. As a result, their function may be better understood and valued. This leads us back to earlier discussions relating to the stigmatizing nature of midwifery work when compared to nursing. These observations are pertinent to consider, as they may explain how cultivating a stronger relationship with nurses may have been advantageous for midwives in the past, and indeed may remain so, particularly in countries where the status of the midwife remains low. The potential stigma of midwifery work is perplexing. Being in attendance at the beginning of life and having responsibility for the safe arrival of the next generation might be assumed to bring with it high levels of respect and admiration for midwives. However, in many cultures childbirth is a taboo topic, and the 'unmentionable' nature of the work frequently 'contaminates' the birth attendant. For example, midwives (*dai*) in Pakistan are considered to be low caste and defiling.[52] The spectre of the handywoman is never far away, as evident in current-day debates about traditional birth attendants in the developing world. Perhaps it is the primal and mysterious nature of childbirth, with its explicit reference to human sexuality and focus on women's bodies, that stigmatizes the work of midwives.

The extent to which both professions can claim occupational authority and responsibility differs. In general, midwives are seen as having greater responsibility, with births being conducted on the midwife's 'own responsibility' rather than being subject to medical authority.[53] In some countries at least, this has led to higher occupational status, which may in turn have fuelled professional rivalries and tribalism. The 1943 Rushcliffe Report made a clear distinction between British nursing and midwifery, recommending higher pay scales for midwives because of their increased responsibility and autonomy.[54] However, this may have been a tactic to flatter midwives and ensure their loyalty in a time of midwifery shortages and high birth rates, rather than any firm acknowledgement of role hierarchy.[55] Midwives argue that they have greater responsibility and autonomy than nurses, and hold dear to the idea of being an 'autonomous practitioner in their own right', although in reality this is rarely achieved in British midwifery. Moreover, it does remain much more likely for British midwives to work in independent practice, providing total care to women with no medical involvement, than nurses. However, the past two decades have seen moves to increase nurses' autonomy, in the form of increasingly specialized roles, such as the advanced nurse practitioner, with these nurses often taking on what were previously medical tasks. The differing scope and focus of nursing and midwifery also affects the potential for task delegation. Broadly speaking, nursing has a history of assigning bedside care to semi-skilled or even unskilled staff, whereas the statutory responsibility of midwives has precluded handing over of care (at least until the early twenty-first century, when the role of Maternity Support Worker was established). Although both professions argue that hands-on care requires the highest skills and knowledge base, in reality those with these high-level skills are more likely to be found in managerial posts than at the bedside. This care deficit has been exacerbated by the removal of students from workforce numbers (it is estimated that prior to Project 2000, 75 per cent of nurses working on the wards were students). Interestingly, the need for 'second-level', less well-trained and inevitably cheaper assistants for both nurses and midwives has featured in the policy reviews of both services throughout the twentieth century.

For both nurses and midwives, doctors are the key other professionals with whom they need to interact. Their relationships with the medical profession differ, and are linked to the notions of responsibility and autonomy. To generalize, nurses, whether they are content with this role or not, are frequently in the position of acting in a support role to doctors, and carrying out treatments prescribed by a doctor. Despite important moves to enhance autonomy via nursing diagnosis and nurse prescribing, most nurses still function to some extent in a support role. Midwives, on the other hand, contest this dynamic and argue that they are doctors' equals, working alongside doctors as experts in normal birth. In reality, many midwives experience this relationship as an ideal rather than reality.

Conclusion

The histories of nursing and midwifery, and in particular their trajectories towards professionalization, reveal a complex web of allegiances, distrust, feuds and cautious reconciliation. The 'tribalism' noted by the Peat Marwick McLintock Committee in 1989[56] remains evident, with nurses exasperated by the phrase 'don't forget the midwives!'[57] and midwives infuriated by the need to prompt nurses to remember that midwifery is a separate profession.[58] The relationship has been shaped by social and political contexts and frequently manipulated for mutual convenience to what best suits the needs of the time, including differing professional interests and personal ambitions.

At times, midwives across the world may have allied themselves with nurses in order to enhance their professional status, increase their 'respectability' and decrease any negative association with the practice of untrained handywomen and granny midwives. And, as we have seen, nurses have also chosen to link with midwives at times when it has suited them, so the courting has not been merely one-sided. There have certainly been some benefits for midwives from collaborating with a much larger professional group, and thus having a stronger voice. But such strategies have their disadvantages: while they may guarantee professional status and a place at the table, this may be at the expense of maintaining a distinctive identity.

The long-standing effects of co-existing as parallel minority and majority professional groups run through the respective histories. Midwifery has struggled to maintain its identity in the face of what is perceived as a constant threat to its unique characteristics, particularly in settings where midwives may find themselves very much in the minority such as academia and policy making. At times midwives have been in danger of defining themselves more in terms of what they are not – that is, they are *not* nurses, they are *not* doctors – rather than in terms of what they are. Nurses, on the other hand, have had sheer numbers on their side. As noted at the beginning, these practical realities can fuel frustrations. Nurses become irritated by a perceived 'politically correct' necessity of adding 'and midwifery' to discussions,[59] while midwives weary of convincing the sister profession that they indeed have a unique and distinctive identity.

The interwoven histories of nurses and midwives mean that tensions, rivalries and allegiances are unlikely to vanish. But acknowledging these histories should enable nurses and midwives to move on from fixed ways of thinking, to develop a discourse which is inclusive and productive, and which pays due respect to each others' cultures and contributions.

Notes

1. I. Norman and P. Griffiths, '. . . And Midwifery: Time for a Parting of the Ways or a Closer Union with Nursing?' *International Journal of Nursing Studies*, 44 (2007) 521–2; D.R. Thompson, R. Watson and S. Stewart, 'Nursing and Midwifery: Time for an Amicable Divorce?' *International Journal of Nursing Studies*, 44 (2007) 523–4; J. Cameron and

J. Taylor, 'Nursing and Midwifery: Re-evaluating the Relationship', *International Journal of Nursing Studies*, 44 (2007) 855–6.

2. R. Mander, 'Extricating Midwifery from the Elephant's Bed', *International Journal of Nursing Studies*, 45 (2008) 649.

3. A. Thompson, 'Establishing the Scope of Practice: Organizing European Midwifery in the Inter-war Years 1919–1938', in H. Marland and A.M. Rafferty (eds), *Midwives, Society and Childbirth: Debates and Controversies in the Modern Period* (London: Routledge, 1997) pp. 14–37.

4. J.E. Thompson, 'Response to Thompson, D., Watson, R. and Stewart, S.: Guest Editorial: Nursing and Midwifery: Time for an Amicable Divorce?' *International Journal of Nursing Studies*, 44 (2007) 651–2.

5. United Nations Population Fund (UNFPA), *The State of the World's Midwifery: Delivering Health, Saving Lives* (New York: UNFPA, 2011).

6. Thompson, 'Response', p. 651.

7. Thompson, 'Establishing', p. 24.

8. Nursing and Midwifery Council, *Statistical Analysis of the Register 1 April 2007 to 31 March 2008*, pp. 10–11, http://www.nmc-uk.org/Documents/Statistical%20analysis%20of%20the%20register/NMC-Statistical-analysis-of-the-register-2007-2008.pdf, accessed 27 May 2011.

9. Thompson, 'Establishing', p. 25.

10. N. Leap and B. Hunter, *The Midwife's Tale* (London: Scarlet Press, 1993) pp. 48–9.

11. F. Nightingale, *Notes on Lying-In Institutions and a Scheme for Training Midwives* (1872), cited in J. Towler and J. Bramall, *Midwives in History and Society* (London: Croom Helm, 1986) p. 158.

12. J. Hannam, 'Rosalind Paget: The Midwife, the Women's Movement and Reform before 1914', in H. Marland and A.M. Rafferty (eds), *Midwives*, pp. 81–101.

13. *Nursing Notes* (December 1906) p. 173, cited in Hannam, 'Rosalind Paget', p. 82.

14. Mander, 'Extricating', p. 649; B. Cowell and D. Wainwright, *Behind the Blue Door: The History of the Royal College of Midwives, 1881–1981* (London: Bailliere Tindall, 1981) pp. 16, 25; J. Donnison, *Midwives and Medical Men: A History of Inter-Professional Rivalries and Women's Rights* (New York: Schocken Books, 1977) pp. 112–113.

15. Donnison, *Midwives*, p. 113.

16. Mander, 'Extricating', p. 649.

17. Donnison, *Midwives*, p. 113.

18. Mander, 'Extricating', p. 649.

19. Cowell and Wainwright, *Behind*.

20. Donnison, *Midwives*.

21. Towler and Bramall, *Midwives*, p. 199.

22. Donnison, *Midwives*.

23. Towler and Bramall, *Midwives*, p. 228.
24. Communications of the Midwives Union, 6 (1932) p. 71, cited in Thompson 'Establishing', p. 29.
25. Leap and Hunter, *Midwife's Tale*, p. 59.
26. J. Campbell, *Reports on the Physical Welfare of Mothers and Children: England and Wales*, Vol. 2: *Midwives and Midwifery* (London: Carnegie Trust, Tinling & Co., 1917) cited in Towler and Bramall, *Midwives*, p. 201.
27. Campbell, *Reports*.
28. Donnison, *Midwives*.
29. Donnison, *Midwives*.
30. R. De Vries and R. Barroso, 'Midwives among the Machines: Re-creating Midwifery in the Late Twentieth Century', in Marland and Rafferty (eds), *Midwives*, pp. 248–72.
31. Thanks are due to Dr Tania McIntosh for discussions about her research in this area, which has been published in her book *A Social History of Maternity Care* (Abingdon, Oxford: Routledge, 2012).
32. J.F. Walker, 'Midwife or Obstetric Nurse? Some Perceptions of Midwives and Obstetricians of the Role of the Midwife', *Journal of Advanced Nursing*, 1 (1976) 129–38.
33. UKCC, *Project 2000: A New Preparation for Practice* (London: UKCC, 1986); UKCC, *Project 2000 and the Midwife* (London: UKCC, 1986).
34. UKCC, *Project 2000: New Preparation*, p. 33, para. 6.
35. J. Greenwood (1985) cited in J. Kent, *Social Perspectives on Pregnancy and Childbirth for Midwives, Nurses and the Caring Professions* (Buckingham: Open University Press: 2000) p. 57.
36. S. Hislop, B. Inglis, P. Cope, B. Stoddart and C. McIntosh, 'Situating Theory in Practice: Student Views of Theory-Practice in Project 2000 Nursing Programmes', *Journal of Advanced Nursing*, 23:1 (1996) 171–7.
37. Kent, *Social Perspectives*.
38. UKCC, *Fitness for Practice: Summary*, Chair: Sir Leonard Peach (London: UKCC, 1999) p. 2.
39. UKCC, *Fitness for Practice*, Chair: Sir Leonard Peach (London: UKCC, 1999).
40. A.R. Hochschild, *The Managed Heart: Commercialisation of Human Feeling* (Berkeley, CA: University of California Press, 1983).
41. B. Hunter, 'Conflicting Ideologies as a Source of Emotion Work in Midwifery', *Midwifery*, 20 (2004) 261–71; W. Duggleby and K. Wright, 'The Hope of Professional Caregivers Caring for Persons at the End of Life', *Journal of Hospice and Palliative Nursing*, 9:1 (2007) 42–9.
42. *Midwifery 2020: Delivering Expectations* (Cambridge: Jill Rogers Association, 2010) http://midwifery2020.org.uk/documents/M2020 Deliveringexpectations-FullReport2.pdf, accessed 21 December 2011.

43. Council of Deans for Health, 'Press Release 2008', http://www.rcn.org. uk/__data/assets/pdf_file/0006/251457/RAE2008CoDpressrelease 081218.pdf, accessed 17 July 2011.
44. Personal communication from NMC and RCM. In 1989, Oxford Brookes began the first degree programme for the pre-registration (direct-entry) midwifery programme. The first degree programme for 18 month (nurse-trained) students commenced in September 1990, and was a joint venture between Kings College, and Queen Charlotte's College of Nursing and Midwifery.
45. J.K. McFarlane, *The Proper Study of the Nurse* (London: Royal College of Nursing, 1970).
46. U. Inman, *Towards a Theory of Nursing* (London: Royal College of Nursing, 1975).
47. R. Weir, *A Leap in the Dark: The Origins and Development of the Department of Nursing Studies, University of Edinburgh* (Cornwall: Jamieson Library of Newmill, 1996).
48. L. Page, 'Professing Midwifery', *Evidence-Based Midwifery*, 7:1 (2009) 4–7.
49. R. Bryar, *Theory for Midwifery Practice* (Basingstoke: Palgrave Macmillan, 1995).
50. C. Rees, 'A Retrospective: Jennifer Sleep's Classic Research Study on the Use of Episiotomy in Labour', *MIDIRS Midwifery Digest*, 17:3 (2007) 319–22.
51. UNFPA, *The State of the World's Midwifery*.
52. K. Bharj, 'Pollution: Midwives Defiling South Asian Women', in M. Kirkham (ed.), *Exploring the Dirty Side of Women's Health* (London: Routledge, 2006) pp. 66–7.
53. De Vries and Barroso, *Midwives*.
54. Ministry of Health, *The Midwives Salaries Committee*, Rushcliffe Report (London: HMSO, 1943).
55. R. Dingwall, A.M. Rafferty and C. Webster, *An Introduction to the Social History of Nursing* (London: Routledge, 1988) p. 168.
56. Peat Marwick McLintock, *Review of the United Kingdom Council and the Four National Boards for Nursing, Midwifery and Health Visiting* (London: HMSO, 1989).
57. Norman and Griffiths, '. . . And Midwifery', p. 521.
58. Cameron and Taylor, 'Nursing and Midwifery'.
59. Norman and Griffiths '. . . And Midwifery', p. 521.

10

Epilogue: Contemporary Challenges

Jane Sandall and Anne Marie Rafferty

This collection of essays has brought together the history of nursing and midwifery in Britain since *c.*1700. The purpose of this end piece is to bring the picture up to date by examining the challenges of the twenty-first century.

One of the advantages of a sociological perspective is that it can provide a critical understanding when we examine social change. The term 'Profession' has been used as a shorthand term for occupational groups who have achieved positions of high status and income in society and whose work is characterized by legally sustained privileges. Using historical sources, sociological writers have explained how professional power and status have been achieved through a process of professionalization, for example by a Weberian process of occupational monopoly and closure.[1] Thus a sociological lens analyses the role of the state in supporting strategies of professionalization, and the role of specialized knowledge in securing and maintaining privileges.

If we apply such an analysis to current issues, the Prime Minister's Commission on Nursing and Midwifery can be seen to address challenges in the following key areas: practice, licensing, education and improving the status of nursing and midwifery in society. Published in 2010, the report on the state of nursing and midwifery in England has been the first overarching review of nursing and midwifery in England since the Committee on Nursing chaired by Asa Briggs, which reported in 1972. The Commission aimed to explore how the nursing and midwifery professions could take a central role in the design and delivery of twenty-first-century ser-vices. It considered all branches of nursing as well as midwifery, in all settings, services and sectors within and outside the NHS.[2] The report responds to policy challenges that include the need to constrain costs against increasing health-care demand, and future 'carequakes' arising from long-term conditions, lifestyle behaviour, obesity, drug and alcohol addiction, the complex needs of ageing and preventing problems in the early years.

The report argues that the public image of nursing is out of date in many ways, and that a new image is required in which nurses are not poorly educated handmaidens to doctors. It argues, firstly, for greater occupational and individual autonomy, for example a lead-ing role for nurses in caring for people with long-term conditions, a named midwife for every woman, and increased managerial and pro-fessional accountability for senior nurses and midwives who would champion quality from the point of care to the Executive Board. The second argument is for protection of the title 'nurse' to nurses registered by the Nursing and Midwifery Council, the regulation of advanced nursing and midwifery practice and the regulation of sup-port workers. Degree-level qualification, a career structure to support work across the full range of health and social care settings and fund-ing for research into the evidence base on the value of nursing and midwifery are also key recommendations.

The report points out that there are well over half a million regis-tered nurses and midwives in England, 90 per cent of them women, plus an unknown and growing number of nursing and maternity sup-port staff. Nursing and midwifery account for a large share of public spending, including over £13bn spent in 2009 on NHS pay and pre-registration education alone. Despite the size of this spend, relatively little is known about its cost-effectiveness. The report also argues that nursing and midwifery degrees are an important route to social mobil-ity: nurses and midwives are often the first person in the family to get a degree, often working-class women, often from black and minority ethnic groups.

The government's response has to be contextualized within chal-lenging financial times. Favour is given to raising the public profile, increasing the scope of nursing practice with the elderly, supporting one-to-one midwifery care and ensuring degree-level registration for all new nurses from 2013. Midwives already have degree-level regis-tration. However, there is no endorsement of regulatory changes or support for advanced practice roles supported by regulation.

Thus, in response to current challenges to the status of nursing and midwifery, the Prime Minister's Report encompasses classic professionalizing strategies of greater occupational autonomy, state support for regulation and protection of function, and upgrading education credentials. It has achieved success in some of these spheres. Previous analyses of nursing and midwifery suggest that regulating entry and calling for a uniform education and state registration have all been credentialist tactics of an exclusionary nature, which aimed to improve the status and training of nurses and midwives pursued by an elite group of practitioners who hoped that state-sponsored registration would transform nursing and midwifery into occupations suitable for 'educated refined gentlewomen'.[3] Dingwall et al.[4] pointed out that there are two other important factors. One is the attitude of service users or patients and the other is the attitude of the state, suggesting that it is these three forces that have shaped the status of nursing and midwifery in the twentieth century.

The current analysis highlights similar challenges facing nursing and midwifery as in the last century and similar tactics to improve the lot of nurses and midwives with some indications of state support for the latest professional project, particularly in achieving graduate registration. Where nursing and midwifery have differed in strategies is that midwifery has focused on the importance of relationships with women, successfully mobilizing women's organizations to support the widening of scope of practice of midwives.[5] In the arena of care relationships, nursing would be wise to think about how the changing nature of health care will increase patient journeys across boundaries and how the key role that nurses can play in care co-ordination may also alter the nature of the relationship between nurses and patients over time.

What we argue here, therefore, is that there is more continuity with the grand challenges that nursing and midwifery experienced in the past than radical change. History provides a useful illustration of how the wider context of change often provides the trigger for policy shifts to happen, but that these are characterized by convergence between the interests of the state and the profession and, not uncommonly, a dollop of luck or contingency.[6] Is it a coincidence that nursing gained degree entry status at a time when the wider policy favoured 40 per cent plus of school leavers entering university? Some strides have been made, yet nursing and midwifery continue to lag behind other professions such as medicine in the development of a career structure with clearly defined progression points. Investment in the post-qualification career structure is haphazard and treated as a dispensable luxury at times of financial pressure. Although the move to degree registration brings England into line with Scotland, Northern Ireland and Wales, change has been hard won and has had a long gestation period since the argument for a degree-based profession was first made in the Judge Report of 1985.[7] Project 2000 UKCC[8] set out to break the apprenticeship system in which students were pairs of hands and education was subordinated to service. Much has been achieved in the interim. However, Project 2000 also recommended the introduction of support workers to fill the vacuum left by students, a recommendation which was not implemented in the headlong rush into higher education. The move to integrated care and the production of a nursing student as capable of working in the community as the acute sector post-qualification remains a work in progress, with the 'big bang' of the move to community yet to happen.

The major stumbling block in education policy remains a credible student support funding system. Nor has the move to degree been without controversy. Remnants of the 'too clever to care debate' continue to reverberate round the columns of Sunday newspapers. The fear remains that recruitment problems will be exacerbated by a significant number of potential students who are appropriately caring, but who lack the necessary academic entry qualifications. Far from being a foreign country, the past provides familiar solutions for current policy challenges, translating a time of pressure into calls to bring back the enrolled nurse, perhaps not literally, but an assistant nurse to be recognized and regulated to fill the 'care' gap. This is reinforced by reports in which higher education is often blamed for the perception that nursing has 'lost its way'. Implicit within this critique is nostalgia for a 'golden age' in which uniforms were starched, patients grateful and nurses knew their place. The power of the image tells us something about the public perception of nursing – not only that it lags behind the reality of nursing work but that it is not a venue for high flyers. The poor image of the profession for school leavers was the starting point for the Briggs Committee.[9] Retro images are reinforced by politicians' desire to 'bring back matron', albeit in an updated form. But the past to which this perception belongs is largely a mythical past. For the history of nursing and midwifery has not been characterized by cocoa, comfort blankets, warm words and a reassuring presence in the face of fear. Rather, it has been characterized by struggle and challenge for recognition of the broad range of skills and capabilities required to provide excellent care across a wide spectrum

of activities ranging from attending to bodily needs to managing complex technologies; providing comfort to interpreting diagnostic data; undertaking research to providing leadership; and influencing policy at the highest levels.[10]
History suggests that nursing has been a divided house but now is the time to put our house in order.[11] It also tells us that poor practice is not a thing of the past. Recent cases demonstrate that rooting out poor practice is our highest priority, especially for the frail elderly and most vulnerable within our society. We need to understand the dynamics that lead to poor care in both nursing and midwifery, and to recognize the sentinel signs which tell us we are heading in that direction and prevent catastrophes of care before they happen. We know the elements of positive practice environments which foster better outcomes for patients and nurses, and for midwives and mothers.[12] Leading by example is the most powerful influence on the behaviour of others. As the histories of nursing and midwifery have shown, clarity of purpose, courage and collaboration with all parts of the system are needed in order to change the experiences of those receiving and those providing care.

Notes

1. G. Larkin, *Occupational Monopoly and Modern Medicine* (London: Tavistock, 1983); E. Friedson, *Profession of Medicine: A Study of Applied Knowledge* (Chicago: University of Chicago Press, 1988); M. Larson, *The Rise of Professionalism* (Berkeley: University of California, 1977).
2. Prime Minister's Commission, *Front Line Care: The Future of Nursing and Midwifery in England*, Report of the Prime Minister's Commission on the Future of Nursing and Midwifery in England (2010), http://webarchive.nationalarchives.gov.uk/20100331110400/http://cnm.independent.gov.uk/the-report/
3. *British Journal Nursing* (1904) p. 992, cited in A. Witz, 'Patriarchy and Professions: The Gendered Politics of Occupational Closure', *Sociology*, 24 (1990) 685.
4. R. Dingwall, A.M. Rafferty and C. Webster, *An Introduction to the Social History of Nursing* (London: Routledge, 1988).
5. J. Sandall, 'Continuity of Midwifery Care in England: A New Professional Project?' *Gender, Work and Organization*, 3:4 (1996) 215; J. Sandall, I.L. Bourgeault, J.M. Wouter and A. Schuecking Beate, 'Deciding Who Cares: Winners and Losers in the Late Twentieth Century', in R. De Vries, C. Benoit, E.R. Van Teijlingen and S. Wrede (eds), *Birth by Design: Pregnancy, Maternity Care, and Midwifery in North America and Europe* (New York and London: Routledge, 2001).

6. A.M. Rafferty and R. Traynor, 'Context, Convergence and Contingency: Political Leadership for Nursing', *Journal of Nursing Management*, 12:4 (July 2004) 258–64.

7. Royal College of Nursing, 'The Education of Nurses: A New Dispensation', Commission on Nursing Education (Judge Report) (London: RCN, 1985).

8. United Kingdom Central Council for Nursing, Midwifery and Health Visiting, 'Project 2000: The Final Proposals', Project Paper 9 (London: UKCC, 1987).

9. *Report of the Committee on Nursing* (Briggs Report) Cmnd.5115 (London: HMSO, 1972) p. 54.

10. A.M. Rafferty, *The Politics of Nursing Knowledge* (London: Routledge, 1986).

11. E. Baer, 'Women and the Politics of Career Development: The Case of Nursing', in A.M. Rafferty, J. Robinson and R. Elkan (eds), *Nursing History and the Politics of Welfare* (London: Routledge, 1997).

12. L.H. Aiken, S.P. Clarke, D.M. Sloane, J. Sochalski and J.H. Silber, 'Hospital Nurse Staffing and Patient Mortality, Nurse Burnout, and Job Dissatisfaction', *Journal of the American Medical Association*, 288:16 (23–30 October 2002) 1987–93; M. Hatem, J. Sandall, D. Devane, H. Soltani and S. Gates (2008) 'Midwife-Led Versus Other Models of Care for Childbearing Women', *The Cochrane Database of Systematic Reviews* (2008: Issue 4), Art. No.: CD004667. DOI: 10.1002/ 14651858.CD004667.pub2.

Recommended Further Reading

Nursing

Abel-Smith, B., *A History of the Nursing Profession* (London: Heinemann, 1960).

Allen, D., *The Changing Shape of Nursing Practice* (London: Routledge, 2001).

Baly, M. (ed.), *Nursing and Social Change*, 3rd edn (London: Routledge, 1995).

Baly, M. and Skeet, M., *A History of Nursing at the Middlesex Hospital, 1747–1990* (London: Middlesex Hospital Nurses' Benevolent Fund, 2000).

Bostridge, M., *Florence Nightingale: The Woman and Her Legend* (London: Viking, 2008).

Boudino, I., Carré, J. and Révauger, C. (eds), *The Invisible Woman: Aspects of Women's Work in Eighteenth-Century Britain* (Aldershot: Ashgate, 2005).

Bradshaw, A., *The Project 2000 Nurse: The Remaking of British General Nursing, 1978–2000* (London: Whurr, 2001).

Brockbank, W., *The History of Nursing at the M.R.I., 1752–1929* (Manchester: Manchester University Press, 1970).

Davies, C., *Gender and the Professional Predicament in Nursing* (Buckingham: Open University Press, 1995).

Davies, C. (ed.), *Rewriting Nursing History* (London: Croom Helm, 1980).

Dingwall, R., Rafferty, A.M. and Webster, C., *An Introduction to the Social History of Nursing* (London: Routledge, 1988).

Hallam, J., *Nursing the Image: Media, Culture and Professional Identity* (London, Routledge, 2000).

Hallett, C.E., *Containing Trauma: Nursing Work in the First World War* (Manchester: Manchester University Press, 2009).

Hawkins, S., *Nursing and Women's Labour in the Nineteenth Century: The Quest for Independence* (London: Routledge, 2010).

Lane, P., Raven, N. and Snell, K.D.M. (eds), *Women, Work and Wages in England, 1600–1850* (Woodbridge: Boydell, 2004).

Maggs, C., *The Origins of General Nursing* (London: Croom Helm, 1983).

McGann, S., Crowther, A., and Dougall, R., *A History of the Royal College of Nursing* (Manchester: Manchester University Press, 2009).

Moore, J., *A Zeal for Responsibility: The Struggle for Professional Nursing in Victorian England, 1868–1883* (Athens: The University of Georgia Press, 1988).

Mortimer, B. and McGann, S. (eds), *New Directions in the History of Nursing* (Abingdon: Routledge, 2005).

Porter, R. (ed.), *Patients and Practitioners: Lay Perceptions of Medicine in Pre-Industrial Society* (Cambridge: Cambridge University Press, 1985).

Rafferty, A.M., *The Politics of Nursing Knowledge* (London: Routledge, 1996).

Robinson, J., *Mary Seacole: The Charismatic Black Nurse Who Became a Heroine of the Crimea* (London: Constable, 2005).

Summers, A., *Angels and Citizens: British Women as Military Nurses 1854–1914* (London: Routledge and Kegan Paul, 1988).

Sweet, H.M. with Dougall, R., *Community Nursing and Primary Healthcare in Twentieth-Century Britain* (Abingdon: Routledge, 2008).

Walby, S., Greenwell, J., Mackay, L. and Soothill, K., *Medicine and Nursing: Professions in a Changing Health Service* (London: Sage, 1994).

Whaley, L., *Women and the Practice of Medical Care in Early Modern Europe, 1400–1800* (Basingstoke: Palgrave Macmillan, 2011).

White, R., *Social Change and the Development of the Nursing Profession. A Study of the Poor Law Nursing Service, 1848–1948* (London: Henry Kimpton, 1978).

White, R., *The Effects of the National Health Service on the Nursing Profession* (London: King's Fund, 1985).

Yeo, G., *Nursing at Bart's: A History of Nurse Service and Nurse Education at St Bartholomew's Hospital, London* (Stroud: Alan Sutton, 1995).

Midwifery

Bashford, A., *Purity and Pollution: Gender, Embodiment and Victorian Medicine* (London: Macmillan Press Ltd., 1998).

Campbell, R. and Macfarlane, A., *Where to be Born? The Debate and the Evidence*, 2nd edition (Oxford: National Perinatal Epidemiology Unit, 1994).

Cody, L.F., *Birthing the Nation: Sex, Science and the Conception of Eighteenth-Century Britons* (Oxford: Oxford University Press, 2005).

Cowell, B. and Wainwright, D., *Behind the Blue Door: The History of the Royal College of Midwives, 1881–1981* (London: Balliere Tindall, 1981).

Evenden, D., *The Midwives of Seventeenth-Century London* (Cambridge and New York: Cambridge University Press, 2000).

Fealy, G.M. (ed.), *Care to Remember: Nursing and Midwifery in Ireland* (Cork: Mercier Press, 2005).

Fildes, V., Marks, L. and Marland, H., *Women and Children First: International Maternal and Infant Welfare, 1870–1945* (London: Routledge, 1992).

Garcia, J.K. and Richards, R.M., *The Politics of Maternity Care: Services for Childbearing Women in the Twentieth Century* (Oxford: Clarendon Press, 1990).

Green, M.H., *Women's Healthcare in the Medieval West: Texts and Contexts* (Aldershot: Ashgate, 2000).

Hunter, L. and Hutton, S. (eds), *Women, Science and Medicine 1500–1700: Mothers and Sisters of the Royal Society* (Stroud: Sutton, 1997).

King, H., *Midwifery, Obstetrics and the Rise of Gynaecology. The Uses of a Sixteenth-Century Compendium* (Aldershot and Burlington, VT: Ashgate, 2007).

Lawrence, S.C., *Charitable Knowledge: Hospital Pupils and Practitioners in Eighteenth-Century London* (Cambridge: Cambridge University Press, 1996).

Leap, N. and Hunter, B., *The Midwife's Tale* (London: Scarlet Press, 1993).

Loudon, I., *Death in Childbirth: An International Study of Maternal Care and Maternal Mortality, 1800–1950* (Oxford: Clarendon Press, 1992).

Marland, H. (ed.), *The Art of Midwifery: Early Modern Midwives in Europe* (London: Routledge, 1993).

Marland, H. and Rafferty, A.M. (eds.), *Midwives, Society and Childbirth: Debates and Controversies in the Modern Period* (London; Routledge, 1997).

Oakley, A., *The Captured Womb* (Oxford: Basil Blackwell, 1984).

Reid, L., *Midwifery in Scotland: A History* (Erskine, Renfrewshire: The Scottish History Press, 2011).

Riska, E. and Wegar, K. (eds), *Gender, Work and Medicine: Women and the Medical Division of Labour* (London: Sage, 1993).

Symonds, A. and Hunt, S.C., *The Midwife and Society* (Basingstoke: Macmillan Press, 1996).

Tew, M., *Safer Childbirth? A Critical History of Maternity Care* (London: Chapman and Hall, 1990).

Towler, J. and Bramall, J., *Midwives in History and Society* (London: Croom Helm, 1986).

Van Teijlingen, E.R., Lowis, G.W., McCaffery, P. and Porter M. (eds), *Midwifery and the Medicalization of Childbirth: Comparative Perspectives* (New York: Nova Science Publishers, 2004).

Williams, A.S., *Women and Childbirth in the Twentieth Century* (Stroud: Sutton Publishing Ltd, 1997).

Wilson, A., *The Making of Man-Midwifery: Childbirth in England, 1660–1770* (Cambridge: Harvard University Press, 1995).

International Comparisons

Buhler-Wilkerson, K., *No Place Like Home: A History of Nursing and Home Care in the United States* (Baltimore: John Hopkins University Press, 2001).

D'Antonio, P., *American Nursing: A History of Knowledge, Authority, and the Meaning of Work* (Baltimore: Johns Hopkins University Press, 2010).

Feldberg, G.D. et al. eds., *Women, Health and Nation: Canada and the United States since 1945* (Montréal: McGill-Queen's University Press, 2003).

Fraser, G.J., *African American Midwifery in the South: Dialogues of Birth, Race, and Memory*, 1st edn (Cambridge, MA: Harvard University Press, 1998).

Goan, M.B., *Mary Breckinridge: The Frontier Nursing Service and Rural Health in Appalachia* (Chapel Hill, NC: University of North Carolina Press, 2008).

Godden, J., *Lucy Osburn, a Lady Displaced: Florence Nightingale's Envoy to Australia*, (Sydney, Australia: Sydney University Press, 2006).

McPherson, K., *Bedside Matters: The Transformation of Canadian Nursing, 1900–1990* (Toronto: University of Toronto Press, 1996).

Mitchinson, W., *Giving Birth in Canada, 1900–1950* (Toronto: University of Toronto Press, 2002).

Smith, S.L. *Japanese American Midwives; Culture, Community, and Health Politics, 1880–1950* (Chicago: University of Illinois Press, 2005).

Ulrich, L.T., *A Midwife's Tale: The Life of Martha Ballard, Based on Her Diary 1785–1812* (New York: Alfred A. Knopf, 1990).

Index